A spectacularly honest insight into c
two of the most inspiring people I kno
even elite fitness Gods suffer the same
mortals and that someday we

Wendy Bodkin - CEO and Athlete

A truly inspirational read. Every page provoked a new thought which challenged my current processes and beliefs creating hundreds of questions inside me of how I should act as coach and leader, as well as how I should approach my own fitness journey. I will be keeping this one in the back pocket to keep reigniting the fire and desire for some time!

James Reddy - Athlete and Coach

I stayed up late last night reading your book as I couldn't put it down. Your book was an eye opener and a great motivational read. It was also an emotional journey as I personally related to a lot of the content (except the 'broom closet', but boy how I laughed 'til I cried). Thank you for inspiring me to find and embrace my hidden athlete.

Crystal Knox - Mother of 4

Amazingly honest and brave. Fitlosphy is incredible. I read it last night and feel so privileged to have received so much wisdom and insight. It's written with such honesty and strength...I couldn't put it down. I love how simple, yet profound Sharny and Julius work is. It's such an honour to read and witness such an incredible journey. Thank you for writing it, sharing your own and your family's lives, and saying what I myself believe. Loved it!

Jamie Milne - Author of 12 Weeks to an Ultramarathon

From the first page, I was hooked! Fitlosophy is a powerful book about the mindset behind personal transformation. It's not only a philosophy but a tactical roadmap for creating a kick-ass body & life. A powerful life starts with a powerful body and Sharny and Julius know how to get you there.

Lyndelle Palmer Clarke - International Bestselling Author of Dailygreatness Journal

FITlosophy

1

Chasing physical perfection in a world of gluttony

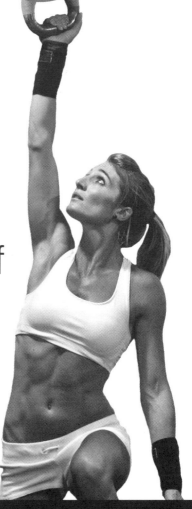

sharnyandjulius™

FITlosophy 1 by **sharnyandjulius**™

chasing physical perfection in a world of gluttony

PO Box 7527
Sippy Downs
QLD 4556
Australia

ABN: 48 016 758 265
www.sharnyandjulius.com
email: info@sharnyandjulius.com

Edited:	Glynny Kieser
Distributor:	berminghambooks.com
Cover Photography:	depositphotos
Typesetting and Design:	sharnyandjulius
ISBN:	978-0-9871428-2-5

Dedication

This book is dedicated to You.

The champion, the athlete, the leader. You were born to change the world, to give simple people like us permission to be better, to try harder, to have a go.

Keep making a difference. Keep chasing perfection. Stay courageous, stay excellent. Stay you.

Thankyou from the bottom of our hearts, you may never know the impact you have in the world, but we will.

sharnyandjuliustm

"Focus on the pursuit of excellence leading to mastery. This should be the purpose of your life, or you could cop out and just choose to be a passenger.

Start on the journey for health mastery and the seeds of excellence will invariably creep into the rest of your life, showing up in unexpected, but remarkable ways."

sharnyandjulius™

Contents

Fat People Have Enough Help

How did it come to this?

Wiping the grimy sweat off his brow with an old rag, the man looks up.

"The wind must be light", he thinks, watching the column of smoke rise up, up, up, out of the cavern, through the circular opening and into the bright blue sky.

It's been a long time since he felt the wind. He wouldn't say it loud, but he's missed it. For the past few months he's caught himself thinking about it more and more often. Nearly two whole hours passed that morning before he rolled out of his cot, drifting in and out of his dreams. Dreams of the past, dreams of adventure.

Now, looking at the wind, he goes there again, this time for real. Shovel clanging to the ground, he steps out of the mud and starts walking. Not looking back, he just keeps walking.

Once he gets to the wall, he begins to climb. It's hard to start, but as he gets higher he drops his bags, one at a time. "Fill your bags, fill your bags" the gold merchant's voices echo through the cavern, "fill your bags with treasure."

I have so many bags, he thinks, letting each one slip off his shoulder, down his arm and into the abyss. He's getting higher now, the mouth of the cavern seems so much bigger, so much brighter.

Crossing out of the shadows and into the light, he hears cries from below. Some of them excited, most of them angry. Again and again, faces from his past flash in front of him.

They're all so sad he thinks, emotions battling inside his chest. A deep driving need pushes him to keep climbing, he *must* climb, but every step is poisoned with guilt.

"Just one look" his heart begs. If he looks back he'll see him, eyes bright, filled with tears. "Daddy, daddy" he'll be crying. "Why are you leaving me!"

On he climbs, desperately wanting to look back, his heart feels like it's tearing into little pieces as he makes out the voice of his son. Daddy, daddy!"

It takes every shred of willpower he has to not turn his head. One look back and it's over. He'll be back in the mud, buried by nightfall.

Higher and higher he climbs, out of the endless cave. "It started with greed," he whispers. "Greed." He can say that here, nobody can hear him. "*Greed*" It feels good to say what he means. "It was *greed* that got you *stuck*." He wickedly enjoys the feeling of the offensive words coming out of his mouth.

Why did they become so offensive? He wonders, thinking back to the landing. Standing on the bow, over a sea of wagons, the captain had declared it the new frontier. "Go forth on the greatest adventure in human history. Never stop exploring!"

The feeling that drove him then, sings painfully in his heart now. "We were never meant to be down here", his fist pounds the cliff face, bleeding finger pointing to the sky, "we're meant to be out there!"

The first few months after the landing were an adventure. Every day was a new discovery. Every sunrise held a mystery, a promise waiting to be explored. A man and his wife pioneering the new frontier together.

It was glorious, it was beautiful, it was simple. It was meant to be forever.

"They need you, you're fast, you're agile, you're light, would you please help them. Please!" The words would haunt him for decades. Turning his wagon around, the man and his wife answered the cry for help, they wanted to help.

Cresting the final hill he saw it, a giant, swollen worm of wagons. "How could they be this far behind?" he wondered. Coming down onto the flats, he found his answer.

From everywhere glistened the brightness of gold. Stocked up in the wagons, in the saddlebags of the horses and in the peoples pockets were piles and piles of the precious metal.

People were scurrying around filling their wagons with gold, in the old world, this would make them all rich. An old preacher was standing on a hill, his eery voice falling on deaf ears. "The old world is gone. Gold is everywhere here, it's not precious, it's worthless."

"We're rich!" cried the people, filling their wagons.

"These people won't listen," said the preacher to the man, "there is more gold here than we've ever found in history. It's poisoning them, it's weighing them down, but still they collect it, stuffing their wagons, now buried to the axles."

"Empty your wagons! Empty your pockets!" tried the man. "I've been to the base of the mountains and beyond. Every hill and every valley is the same, this place glistens with gold, we will never run out"

But nobody believed him. "If we can just get their wagons moving, they can see for themselves," thinks the man, grabbing a shovel.

And so began the great dig. "Your wagons are too fat and slow", the man cried, back bent, hands bleeding.

"Our wagons have big frames" they said, and for a while he believed them, always trying to help. But once there was no space left in the wagons, and the people threw out their children to help dig, he knew it wasn't the wagons.

"Throw out some of your gold!" the man said.

"Dig faster!" the people would reply. So the man dug.
"Your wagons are too heavy, throw out some of your gold," he tried.

"It's not our fault, it's the gold merchants, they can manufacture it for cheaper than we can get it ourselves!"

"It's junk gold," the man replied, "you don't need that much!"

"But it's so cheap" they'd say. Not wanting to leave their treasure alone, they traded parts of their wagons for bigger piles of gold.

Gold was everywhere, it was crushing the backs of the horses and weighing down the people. "If everybody has so much gold, it's worthless!" cried the man, the axles on his own wagon collapsing under the weight of his wife's gold.

Looking up, he could see her, overcome by greed. Nestled in her arms, surrounded by gold, was his boy. Born into this world of greed, what hope would he have of adventure?

"Dig us out honey," said his wife. "Dig us out and we can be on our way."

"Lose some of the gold," he pleaded.

"It's not the gold, it's the witchdoctors," she replied. "They have pretended to help us, giving our horses pills to help their weak hearts. But the pills have side effects; the horses act strange. The witchdoctors are now selling us pills to help with the side effects, but the new pills have other side effects"

"It's not the witch doctors fault that our wagon is stuck," pleaded the man.

"We've heard from the experts, and listened to their lessons, we just need to oil our axles and dig ourselves out. As soon as we fix our wheels, we'll get going."

Looking sadly up at the woman who loved him, the man continued digging.

The next few years were a blur. Dig, dig, dig, always wanting to help.

Back on the slope, the man thinks about his wife, barely recognisable now, behind her layers and layers of gold. "I can't help them any more," he thinks, turning back to the sky. "They have their unions, they have their support groups, they have their pills and potions, they have enough help."

Fumbling through his pockets, finding gold he must have put there years ago, he thinks about the angry words of his wife. "You're just like us now, you've spent so much time trying to help us that you've become one of us. You're *stuck* too!"

That was last night; his son's birthday. The boy's face, mostly hidden behind his pile of gold would never feel the pleasure of the sun on his back, or the wind in his hair. Giving him his present, a bag of gold, the man had turned to his wife, and in his anger said "look at him, he's *stuck*! It's all your fault!"

Tears stream down his face as he moves on. He can feel the eyes of his wife and son watching his back, hopelessly watching as he abandons them. "I'm sorry" bubbles out of his mouth as he scrambles up the slippery slope.

Finally, he crests the edge of the cavern. Slumping down onto his back, bathed in full sunlight, he begins to sob. "I've left them behind, I'm the worst person ever. I have to go back." The pain in his heart is too much to bear. "Why did I even do this," he cries, "why can't I just be normal like them!"

A distant sound enters his consciousness. It's the voice of his son, carried all the way up here.

"Daddy, daddy."

"I'm coming," he gives up, pocketing a handful of gold. "I'm bringing you a surprise," he cries, forlorn body shuddering with huge sobs.

"Daddy, daddy!" the boy's voice pierces his heart.

"It's lonely out here without you" the man yells, squinting in the sunlight, "I'm coming back!"

"Daddy, daddy!" The echo of his son's voice rattles through his brain. "How could I abandon them!" Crying out at the sky, overcome with emotion he slumps forward and crawls toward the mouth of the great cave.

"DADDY!"

He blinks away the pain.

"DADDY!"

Too afraid to open his eyes, he pushes his head over the edge, toward the sound of the little voice.

"DADDY...

...we did it!"

Little arms wrap tightly around his neck as he hears the words.

"You just had to show us," the voice of his wife sounds different, melodical, joyful even. He opens his eyes to see them both there, perfect skins reflecting the bright midday sun.

"What about the gold?" he asks

"That junk? We don't need that junk, we left it on the slopes"

Tears sting his eyes as he embraces his family, "I'm so sorry for abandoning you."

"You didn't abandon us honey," says his wife, "you *inspired* us."

Looking around, they notice more and more people climbing out of the hole, tattered, torn and bruised, but carrying no junk. Possibility shines out of their eyes, brighter than gold, brighter than diamonds.

Blinking tears away from his eyes, he embraces his family one more time, before turning to face the mountains. "I forgot how perfect this could be," he whispers, "we're perfect." Excitement fills him and spills out like firecrackers. Squeezing the hands of his loved ones, he leaps forward, light as a feather, and with the grace of a leopard, runs off into the meadows with them, strong bodies already beginning to tan.

If there are no stars in the sky, what will we all have to look up to?

This book is for the adventurers, the ones who know that there is more to fitness than losing weight. The ones who know that there is more to life than fitting in, than being normal. You are the inspirers, the leaders.

No longer should you feel guilty when a workmate asks about your exercise blistered hands, no longer should you feel ashamed about what or how little you eat, or wearing tight clothing. No longer can your energy be held in check by society's fat expectations.

You, my friend are a leader. A leader cannot lead from the middle of the pack. Turn around, you must turn your back on them if you love them. You cannot help people by becoming one of them. You must run ahead, you are their beacon of possibility.

People don't need help. They need inspiration. Society has worked so hard to close the gap of equality, all the while sacrificing the growth of humanity.

Until now, we have kept the gap closed by holding back the front runners. Until now, leaders have been ashamed to stand out for what they believe in. Until now, we have dug holes in the dark.

Release your shackles, feel no guilt. Run, swim, play, climb, be perfect in your health and do it proudly. We need you to open the gap, the gap between fat and fit. By doing so, fat people won't feel normal any more, and will be drawn to closing the gap themselves.

Then, because of you being what you were born to be, you will reverse this cancerous plague of obesity and blame gripping our world.

Go forth, great adventurer, as you climb your own cavern, this book shall be your guide and friend.

And from there?

As you charge off alone into the light, don't feel lonely, for following in your footsteps right behind you are the people who love you.

...the world will follow you.

A Bag Of Seeds

Michael Legless was an 18th Century peasant. Born without the use of his legs, he spent the first 23 years of his life in a hand cart drawn by his brother, James.

One day, while rolling through the market quarter of the town, he announced to his brother in the most unexpected voice, "Out of the way, James!"

Stunned by the powerful tone in Michael's usually meek voice, James lowers the handles of the cart and stands aside to see what the fuss is about.

A collective gasp erupts from the marketplace as Michael miraculously climbs out of his seat and as though he'd been doing it his entire life, strides out into the crowd and disappears... seemingly forever.

A few months later, while plouging the field, James stands up to stretch his back. Walking toward him on the trail is a knight, dressed in full chain mail and leading a powerful horse.

"James!" announces the knight in a familiar voice.

"Michael!" calls out a shocked James, "what happened to you?"

"I became a knight!"

"How?" asks a bewildered James.

"Well, do you remember when we were boys how we used to watch the knights ride through our fields, and for the rest of the day you would run around with your wooden sword, fighting all the bushes?"

"Yes."

"Well, a few months ago, I was waiting for you to get back from the quarters, when I saw one of those knights walked past, on some important duty. For the first time ever, I thought to myself *that'd be nice.*

Then a few months later, I saw another one, this time leading a horse, and I thought to myself again, *that'd be nice.*

So then a couple of weeks pass and I see a group of knights marching through the markets. That feeling comes back, this time stronger. I think to myself *that'd be nice*, but this time, I think about it for about an hour.

The next day, I think about it again, and start to see in my head a picture of me walking. *That'd be nice* I say to myself, day dreaming of walking through the park with my own war horse.

Over the next few weeks, the thoughts got stronger and stronger, closer and closer together and lasted longer and longer.

You see, all my life I never did anything about it, never tried, never even thought to try. On the day that I stood up and walked, I woke up thinking about it, and for the whole morning, it was the only thing I could think about. By the time I got to the markets, I just... had to stand up.

So, I stood up.

It's just that simple."

And it is.

It's the same way we all buy cars. It starts as a simple, innocent *that'd be nice*, as we drive past one on the motorway.   Six months later, we notice another one, and think again, *that'd be nice*. A month later, we see another and think *that'd be nice to have*.

A week later, we see another, and 'that'd be nice to have' becomes a lingering thought. The thought lasts longer and longer, and we begin seeing the car more and more, until one day, it is all we can think about, and it seems that it is all we can see. On that day, we go in and test drive the car.

It starts with a just a small seed.

This book is a collection of seeds. We have no illusions of changing the world, we are not elite athletes, we are not humanitarian leaders, we are not politicians. Our job is to simply tell the story and sow the seeds, so that they may one day be picked up and grown in greater people than us.

You, perhaps?

Not all the stories will pertain to you, maybe only one... for now. Whatever you get out of this book is what you are meant to get out of this book.

Sit back, relax... clear your mind, because you're about to go on a magical journey. A journey where you are the hero, and your only duty? Let the stories take your mind where it needs to go.

The rest?

Well.. the rest is up to you.

Selfish Is Generous

6.25pm Tuesday afternoon. The kids have had their milk, read their story and peace descends upon our house. The chill of the evening has not set in yet as we sit out on our deck, listening to the final whip-cracks of the lyrebird in the forest. We watch silently as the moon, big enough to touch, greets us through the trees. As the deep red of the sunset finally gives way to the silvers of the moonlit night, we look to one another.

We've never been apart since the day we first met, eyes locking across a dance floor, we both felt then the pull of fate. And now, sitting next to one another in the silvery darkness, we both know exactly what the other is thinking. We could see it in each other's eyes, the gratitude shines bright, brighter than the moon.

"We've come a long way," says Julius softly, thinking about the journey that has led us to this. "Did you ever imagine, all those years ago, that your life would amount to this?"

"It's gone so quickly, hasn't it" I mumble, drifting off blissfully into day dreams of reminiscence. Growing up in relative poverty, I dreamed of one day living in a big house, with a pool, close to the ocean, surrounded by people who love me and celebrate me. I think back to the little girl who weeped silently at night, the stinging words of her uncle repeating over and over in her head.

"Why don't you come back down to earth with the rest of us, you're never

going to amount to much, so stop chasing selfish dreams"

I wonder what I'd say to that little girl now, would she believe me if I tell her that the house she so vividly dreams about will one day fit on the verandah of where she actually lives, in her private mansion with her own driveway behind enormous electric gates, a huge pool, a tennis court and basketball court as well as the magnificent forest, complete with its own river.

Would she believe me if I told her about her beautiful children and her loving, sexy husband. How would I tell her that one day she will be surrounded by famous, wealthy, influential people, all who love her, all who celebrate her. Would I tell her that all this would be possible, what would I say?

The piercing 'rrrrrring' of our phone cuts my thought pattern before I can answer. Julius answers as I look at the time, 6.35; he's meant to be downstairs in the gym with Aaron. Filing the question away for later, I follow Julius inside.

"You're what? I can't really hear you, it sounds like you're far away"

His powerful frame blocks the doorway. I can't help but snigger as I remember him telling me how his father hated him playing in the hallways or doorways at home - something he would then do on purpose, the cheeky boy.

He was a different type of problem child to me. Gifted with such a high IQ that it would be retested twice, and a natural athleticism that would see him picked for every rep sport he tried, his only failing was his desperation to be normal.

Everything he has ever done has come naturally to him, to the frustration of all around him, he would excel at anything he tried, but the more excited his coaches, teachers and parents would be, the more he felt ostracised and different.

And just like that he'd quit, moving on to the next thing, desperately seeking something that was hard for him, so he could be normal.

He's never spoken to anybody else about this, but it is what still drives him today. Where others in his past have labelled him as anti establishment, or anti authority, lazy or a quitter, I know the truth of it.

He has squandered opportunities, yes, but without that regret, he wouldn't be the thought leader he is today. Terrified of being boxed in, or labelled, or owned, he has sought ways to express himself honestly and completely.

His life purpose now, is to facilitate the greatness in others. As I ponder his remarkable combination of emotional intelligence, artistic brilliance and his calculated, analytical approach to life, he spins on his heels, and without even thinking, glides around me like a panther. *He should have run straight into me* I think, as I hear his voice, shouting this time

"You're where?"

"You're *here*?"

"You're in the *air*?"

"Really! OK, I will"

"Sharn, you're not going to believe this," the excitement in his face is infectious as he throws me the phone. "Stay here" he yells, running out onto the grounds.

I don't have to wonder for long, the low thump, thump, thump grows deafening as a white helicopter just appears from behind the trees. My clothes push tight onto my skin and my eyes water as I try to work out what is going on.

As I squint at the helicopter, a side door opens and there in front of me is Aaron, close enough to see the cheeky grin on his face as he flips me a quick wave.

There is no way anyone can land on a tennis court I think, as Aaron throws out a ladder. Julius is there, directly underneath it, catching the last rungs. I cannot believe my eyes. Aaron Blackman, CEO of one of the fastest growing Australian companies of all time, dressed in a corporate suit, with a gym bag hanging from his shoulder is climbing down a rope ladder, suspended from a helicopter, held on the end by my husband.

I could never explain this to that little girl, all those years ago I think as I run inside, shutting all the windows so the kids don't wake up. Too late, Alexis has climbed out of her cot and is clutching my leg. I swoop her up and run to the window to show her the "pellypoppa." She looks on in wide eyed amazement as the door shuts and the chopper roars away into the night.

The noise of the engines is still thup, thup, thupping in my head as I carry her downstairs. "Wow," is all I can muster when I finally come face to face with the two wide eyed boys. Aaron was not born into wealth, the son of a police officer and nurse, he lives a life underpinned by the need to serve others.

Most business people are seen as greedy and self serving. Outwardly, it would appear that way for Aaron too, but being blessed to know him has allowed us a glimpse at the private life of a super wealthy, high achiever.

Aaron isn't driven by a desire to be rich, he is driven by a desire to help as many people as he can, from his family, to his employees and his clients. While he may be a hard task master, everybody knows that they are in his life because he cares for them. He loves people and feels a responsibility for them, born from the values of his parents.

"I'm so sorry for waking the kids Sharny," he says, the 'aliveness' beaming through his eyes as he reaches out to give Alexis a reassuring pat on the leg. "I just cannot miss my sessions here," he says.

"Wow," I stutter again, thoughts crashing into one another in my head.

"No, I'm serious," he says, "if I don't do my fitness session here, I can't perform at work. If I can't perform at work, then my business suffers, if my business suffers, my employees suffer and I end up spending more time at work, and my family suffers."

I must have still had a look of incredulation on my face, because he clarified even more;

"People see it as selfish, maybe, well I guess it is, I spent a lot of money getting here tonight, and I battle to get here every time, sometimes I have to run out of the office, rudely ignoring everybody so they don't get a chance to ask me any questions, just to get here."

"But I know, and I'm sure they know now because of how often I do it, that if it wasn't for my commitment to fitness, I would not be able to sustain the energy required to run that enormous company, to keep so many people in work, and my family wouldn't have the lifestyle they are used to now. They wouldn't even see me. So I guess, me being selfish is actually me being generous."

And there it was. Emotions flooded through me as I hugged him, Alexis must have felt the moment too, because she put her little arms around him, saying in her sweet voice "cuggle Aawon".

What would I say to that little girl, all those years ago, sobbing into the pillow:

"Leaders must look after themselves first... Selfish is generous."

Quit Guilt

Julius' brother Daniel is in corporate finance. Every time we see him, we want to know what shares to buy that will make us rich. His answer is always "what pill can I take to make me thin?"

We get asked all the time, "what's the one thing I can do right now, that will make the biggest difference."

It's a great question, highlighting people's need for an instantaneous solution. We live in the speed of information age, where answers are found at the push of a button. It is the question that drives the entire fitness and wellness economy, and depending on who you ask, the answers are always different. It's the 'magic pill' question.

If we discovered a magic pill that could miraculously stop you from overeating, give you motivation to exercise and love it, could help drop kilos miraculously, could make you more attractive, magnetic, charismatic, exciting and arousing to be around. A pill that taken once a day, could make you into the person you wished you were, the person you secretly know you should be, trim, tight, toned; a person who lets nothing get in their way, would you take it? Would you buy it?

We've actually found the pill, we've given it to hundreds of people and every single one of them has achieved amazing results, not only physically, but mentally, emotionally and spiritually. We certainly didn't create it, and we don't talk about it enough, but we'll tell you about it right now. But first, a story.

When we first started working together, we used to battle. We were two strong headed people with completely different backgrounds, coming together to run the same business.

We spent a lot of time and money getting better and better at fitness and business, but we could never really take big enough leaps ahead because we would argue about implementation.

We had the same ideas, and the same purpose, it's just that every time we would be ready to push the 'go' button, we'd argue about who should do it, how to do it, and whose idea it was to do it.

If you're married, you'll understand, if you're about to get married, then this is kind of how it goes after the honeymoon period *unless you do something about it*.

If it wasn't for one of our clients at the time, we would probably still be retarding ourselves with arguments about the minutia. Ross told us to go to a thing called Landmark Forum. We nearly didn't go, because Julius hated "make believe woo woo stuff".

Landmark Forum, for those who haven't been is a 3 day seminar in which attendees leave on day 3 with a 'blank canvas'. All the rubbish they have been holding onto their entire lives is put in the past where it belongs, never to affect the future again. It is a remarkable event, and one that has been credited with freeing some of the greatest minds of our time.

Through the course of *the forum*, people get a chance to stand up on stage with the leader while the rest of the participants (around 1,000) watch as they somewhat miraculously release their past.

It is such an intense, interesting and revealing exercise - drug addicts, alcoholics, problem gamblers and criminals talk about and release their past alongside mums and dads who can't talk to their kids or teenagers who are really, really shy.

One of the profound stories, stands out the most.

René [*name changed for privacy*] was a chain smoking overweight heroin junkie. A complete juxtaposition. Most heroin junkies are malnourished and gaunt. But not René. René was enormous. She must have weighed over 220kg, and was shorter than most women.

When René got on stage on the second morning of *the forum*, she told a story of gluttony and excess that unfolded over 22 years of her 29 year life. René was single, couldn't get a job, and was most afraid of becoming a mother one day, but really wanted nothing more than to have kids.

René was the embodiment of sadness. It was in everything about her, the clothes, the stature, the tone of her voice. The people in the front rows wept silently as she told of a childhood of physical and sexual abuse at the hands of her own father.

She told stories of how her father would come home drunk early Saturday mornings and beat her mother, how she would stuff her ears with toilet paper to block the horrific sound of her mother's screams, interrupted by the wet thump, thump of fists meeting face.

René was terrified of her father, but loved her mother. The young five year old wanted only for her parents to love each other.

René knew what would happen to herself if she went downstairs, it had been happening for as long as she could remember.

The love and devotion the young five year old had for her mother was stronger than her immense fear, so every night she would calm her sobbing and dry her eyes, stopping only for a moment to take out her makeshift earplugs before entering the room.

The poor girl would take only a few steps before the attention of her violent father would turn on her, and she would be frozen in place with fear.

In her young mind, she just wanted to say "please stop hurting us daddy," but fear paralysed her tongue. The words died in her mouth.

René couldn't remember a time in her childhood where she was not bruised or bleeding. Her mum begged her to stay inside, because if someone saw her bruises, they would take her away. At the age of 7, fear of another beating and rape became overwhelming. René ran away from home.

It was a Friday night, so she knew her father would not be home for hours. She ran and ran and ran as far as she could, determined to get away, crying the whole time.

She wandered the streets of South Auckland for months, scavenging from rubbish bins and begging for food. She slept on a ledge under the Mangere bridge, stuffing her clothes with old plastic bags to keep warm.

Longing for the embrace of her gentle mother, she cried herself to sleep every night desperately wanting to go home, but too scared to even look in the direction.

Fast forward through a life of petty theft, prostitution and heroin addiction. Somehow, the 29 year old's journey had led her here. Standing in front of the crowd, she told us all how she had spent the last 22 years living on the streets, eating to excess and shooting up heroin.

By the time she finished her story, there was not a dry eye in the place. Silent tension enveloped the hall as we all wondered what next.

"What would you like to say to your parents now?" whispered the forum leader into the microphone.

Nobody breathed as we watched her lean into the microphone, deep eyes staring blankly into history. With a voice of a young child, she whimpered "I'm sorry".

The room exploded in a frenzy of voices. Loud sobbing could be heard through cries of outrage, people were standing up in their seats. The young voice, amplified by the microphone could barely be heard through the din.

"I'm so sorry for leaving you."

And there it was. Guilt. After the crowd had been settled, through some delicate questioning, René came to see that her life was dictated by guilt. Unfounded guilt, but guilt all the same.

Guilt is like a black hole of destruction. It was because of a 5 year old's feelings of guilt that René had stayed so close to home for so long. Guilt that had led her to drugs, it was because of guilt that she ate to excess and beyond. But what was most remarkable about her experience was when she was discussing her heroin and food addictions.

She said that she didn't even like heroin, she hated being fat, didn't even like food and had tried to quit both so many times. Every time coming back to the familiarity.

Why?

Because she would think about the last time she ate to excess or shot up, and would feel guilt. Her guilt would make her eat, and guilt over her eating would make her eat more and more before she got so wound up that she needed a release, and would shoot up heroin.

Six years after the Forum, we ran into René. Unrecognisable, she stopped to chat at the steps to the beach in Mooloolaba, where we live. We couldn't believe it was her. She was thin, she was wearing a bikini.

She told us that she was just up on the coast with her husband and baby daughters, celebrating her graduation from law school. Happiness beamed from her eyes when we asked her what had happened since Landmark.

"I quit."

"I quit guilt," she said. "Heroin, food, alcohol, cigarettes, prostitution; they were what I used to fill the hole that guilt created in me. Landmark helped me quit feeling guilty, and since that day on stage, I've never touched cigarettes, alcohol, heroin or junk food. I'm free.

An absolutely remarkable story, and one that we are privileged to have witnessed first hand. Knowing René has helped us come to realise the power we give to our guilt.

Guilt is not even real. It is a chain we carry on our backs that we put there ourselves. We carry our guilt for years and years rather than casting it off and moving on, we give our guilt power.

Here's an affirmation you can say to yourself if you find yourself holding onto guilt. Just imagine yourself removing big chains off your back as you say the following words out loud:

I did what I did, because I did what I did;
nobody is to blame and I'll serve no penance,
for I will give no power to guilt.

You, Athlete

A swimmers workday is a mind numbing churn of lap after lap after lap in the pool. Physical exhaustion combines with a 'knowing too much about yourself' feeling from spending so much time with only your thoughts for company.

Sport is a job, and swimmers are some of the lowest paid. It is equivalent to manual labour, chain gang stuff. These guys earn a pitiful living, work harder than most athletes, in the most opressive of environments and have nobody to blame for failure other than themselves.

If we coach an athlete through a gym session, we are able to give them instant feedback for style and technique correction. Not so in swimming. Once a swimmer hits the water, there is nothing but splashing and the rhythm of their breathing to keep them company...

And the voices inside their heads.

We have a client who is a logger. You would be very safe to think that a logger would be really, really dumb. He even tells us that when he first met his wife, her mother said "oh no, not a *dumb* logger."

But Ben Douglas [*name changed for privacy*], logger from Gympie, Australia would have to be one of the most analytical, intelligent people we have ever met.

What else can he do when he has to spend 10 hours a day holding a chainsaw with ear muffs on? He thinks. He's living with the voice inside his head.

And to meet Ben, you would think he were a modern day Napoleon. Ben knows himself better than anyone else knows themselves. Ben has spent the last 30 years digesting his weekend's battles slowly and methodically with his hands busy and his ears blocked.

Imagine what you could know if you had 50 hours of alone time.

Gympie is an interesting town in that the passion is squash. Other towns have their football teams, but in the heart of Gympie is their squash club. It's what they do.

Ben loves squash. It is his obsession. Pair an obsession for squash with 50 hours of alone time and you get some serious passion. And knowledge. No, knowing.

Ben knows himself, but more importantly, Ben knows his opponents. He is a one man video analyst. He spends all week remembering the weekend's games. He analyses every shot, he thinks about his strategy and he even talks to us about his *default plays*, something we thought was our closely guarded secret.

Ben understands through his time alone that it's not what you do exceptionally that wins you games, it is your default plays. This is something we work really hard to instil into our athletes. A default play is what you default to when you are exhausted or stressed. It is instinctual, it is a reaction, it is thoughtless. It just happens.

Part of our success with athletes comes from training their default plays. In rugby players for example, we train their proprioception in such a way that even at the end of 80 minutes, when they have run out of fuel, run out of energy and are mentally exhausted, they can, without thinking, tackle with perfect technique.

If you are a rugby person you will know that many games are won in the last 5 minutes of the halves, when the defense is exhausted and making mistakes.

Increased comparative fitness can go a long way to mitigating that risk for a team, but what happens if the game is close and both teams are at their peak fitness?

Default plays. What you do when you can't think.

Understanding this has allowed the players and teams we have coached to feel less stressed in the dying stages, and the results have backed up our instincts. This changes the 'luck' factor in sports.

If a coach knows his default plays, he can coach around them. He can build a game plan around the first 30 minutes, knowing that his players' default will kick in somewhere in the last 10 minutes.

While the opposition is expending a lot of emotional energy and stress in the last 10 minutes, our teams are slotting into their defaults. They head into half time with less emotional energy spent, they essentially have a longer half time break.

Where it gets really, really interesting is when we reprogram someone's default play. Which is what Ben, the logger from Gympie Australia has done to himself, *and knows it.*

Ben has become a master of the default play. He has beaten much better opponents by what he calls his mind games. There are a few of them (and we've translated some excellent ones to other sports - because you can't revolutionise a sport from within), but this is the one that is important for this chapter.

Ben has reprogrammed one of his default plays to a 3 shot winning combination that would make a chess master proud. He can feel when his exhaustion is causing him to lose concentration, and instead of stressing and willing more from himself, he becomes comfortable, familiar even.

A look of serenity glides over his face (also a mind game), his breathing steadies and he relaxes. Playing simple shots, he purposefully leans too far to the left of the court - waiting for his opponent to see the opening and play a fast tight winning shot to Ben's right.

Click, whirrr. Like a tape player, Ben pushes play on his 3 shot default play.

Shot one is a full length stretch that nobody should hit, let alone a 47 year old. Ben's opponent has to scramble to return the fluke shot, running in front of him as he exits his remarkable lunge.

Ben's not even thinking now, he is just dancing. Dancing a dance he has programmed into his mind. Shot 2 of the 3 shot combo is a display of dexterity, what Ben call's his 'tap on the head'. To the opponent, Ben has just executed his second miracle shot.

But it ain't no miracle, it is Ben's well executed and well practiced plan. He has replayed this scenario hundreds of thousands of times in his mind. He is the conductor in the orchestra and the two bodies on court are playing perfectly in tune.

What is amazing is that Ben is not only playing his default play, he is making the opposition play theirs.

He's getting them to show all their cards. Miracle shot 3, if it ever gets there, is a gentle shot, an unbeatable gentle shot that Ben makes look easy, effortless even.

After this default play, Ben knows he has won. He has his opposition burning through emotional fuel so fast that he can just sit back comfortably, and wait for mistakes.

Ben's mind games have allowed him to beat countless more talented players. Younger, fitter and faster.

All self taught, never coached. Not bad for a "dumb" logger?

There is a lot to learn from this story; default plays, coaching and implementing them could fill an entire book on their own, but what we want you to understand is that you can never, ever underestimate the intelligence, self analysis and cunning of loners... And there is no lonelier sport than swimming.

Meet Geoff Huegill.

After an illustrious swimming career, with 2 Olympic medals, 8

Commonwealth medals and a world record to his name, Geoff Huegill retires.

Being out of the pool, Geoff's energy consumption dropped considerably. To give you an idea, swimmers eat twice our daily calories in each meal. That means that for breakfast, they must eat what you will eat over the next 2 days.

Imagine what would happen to you if you ate that much. Well, you don't have to imagine, just google 'Geoff Huegill Fat' and you'll get the idea. He ballooned. He became obese. Previously a svelte, trim athlete, Geoff really let himself go.

He spent a few years like this, under the radar, just eating and working. If you had met him for the first time during these years, you would have never imagined him as an athlete.

But through all that time in the pool, alone with his thoughts Geoff had come to understand himself. You see, most people have played some kind of sport as a child, so have that inherent athleticism, then when family and work pressures get in the way of exercise they balloon, just like Geoff. They're no different to Geoff. They stopped playing sport, ate more than they needed and got fat.

But Geoff did something most people thought impossible. While everybody had accepted him as fat, Geoff held onto his internal 'knowing' that he was an athlete. He was not a fat man needing to lose weight, he was an athlete who had let himself go.

In the following months, Geoff lost over 45 kilograms and remarkably regained his spot on the Australian Commonwealth swim team, winning a gold medal and a commonwealth record.

If it weren't for Geoff's belief that he was an athlete, he would still be shopping for size XXXL. For the fat man or fat woman, it is a simple change of mindset.

I am an athlete.

If someone sees themselves as a fat person, trying to lose weight, they will always be a fat person - no matter how much weight they lose - because that is their default play. If you see yourself as an athlete, then exercise and fitness will be your default play.

Even if you are massively overweight now like Geoff Huegill was then, it's only going to be a matter of time before you want to be yourself again, shed the winter coat and get back in the pool.

A rock, lying immobile in a riverbed for years, becomes covered in moss. Is it still a rock, or is it moss?

Never, ever let anyone you love tell themselves they are fat again. Fat is inactive tissue. Look in the mirror and see only active tissue. Muscle, bones, skin, organs, eyes etc; that is you...

The fat? that's not you, you can't own that.

You are the athlete underneath.

Food Is A Drug That Cannot Be Escaped

Sharny has a friend that I am convinced hates me.

On the outside, Rachael is a beautiful, kind, loving woman. She's the type of girl who will offer to babysit our kids so we can have a night out. She cleaned our house once for us while we were away and remembers all the kid's birthdays. She volunteers at the animal shelter, and I've seen her hand raise a chick that had fallen from its nest.

Sounds like a nice girl right?

Yeah. That's what Sharny keeps telling me. But Rachael keeps throwing my life into turmoil.

Whenever she visits, she brings too much food. Her favourite trick, I'm convinced she does on purpose, much to the disgust of my wife, is to open an enormous box of chocolates, and eat none.

Surely she knows, by the bareness of our cupboards, that a box of chocolates, no matter how big, will not last the night. It's a cruel trick, like opening a bottle of Pinot at an AA meeting.

Sharny defends Rach, saying that she shows love with food.

Rachael came to visit yesterday. Normally I'm forewarned about her visits and make a good excuse to not be there, but she'd been away in Switzerland so Sharny thought it would be rude of me to not be there.

"10 O'clock exactly" I grumble to Sharny, flicking my eyebrows toward the clock. "Like a Stepford Wife" I add quietly, earning myself a stern glare as we walk to the door.

"Maybe I can leave and she can clean the house again. Sniff my undies. Make a doll out of my hair?"

"Behave!"

"I'll do the night feeds for a whole month" Sharny can see my desperation, a ray of hope glimmers in me as I see the puzzled look in her eyes.

A whole month of night feeds is a lot to offer, normally we take a night each, but a whole month of uninterrupted sleep? I can see the puzzled look turn to amazement and she quickly begins to nod.

I turn on my heel and am half way down the hallway at a full sprint when I hear the door creak open. Jumping through the first door I can, I shut it behind me and steady my breathing.

"Shit, shit shit!" In my desperation I jumped into the mop cupboard. "It's alright," I say to myself, slowing my near frantic breathing. "It's alright..."

Before she came, I planned all sorts of reasons to leave and break up the conversation. I set the phone alarm to the same as the ring tone, so I could pretend to get a phone call. I held in my ablutions so I could be forced to go do that and lied to Sharny that I had just changed the kids nappies.

Ignoring the muffled welcome noises, I scan my surroundings. The light from under the door is just enough to make out the mop, the vacuum and the bucket. My right foot is wedged between the vacuum and the mop bucket, forcing me to put all my weight awkwardly on my left leg.

As I slowly reposition my foot, being very careful not to bump the bucket, I realise that I am in fact, fucked.

The poo I had been holding in decided that it was now time to drop into the final passage. It wanted out.

I'm not the sort of guy who can sit on a toilet for hours reading a book. I prefer to spend as little time on the throne as possible, so always wait until last minute. Something that has caught me out in my younger years. Something that is threatening to ruin my day right now.

"Think, think, think, think, think." My hands are sweating. "*It's so fucking hot in here*" I spit, jaw clenched shut. Something poking into my back is starting to burn. If I move fast, I'll make a racket, or shit my pants. I slowly try to move away as I realise what it is.

The exit pipe of the hot water cylinder is branding me between the shoulders, but I can't move away because of the angle I'm holding. Sweat beading down my forehead I go the only way I can. Down. Crouching slowly I eventually escape the pain. I wonder about the weird shape the burn will have, as my thighs begin to quiver.

The mumbling of the girls is getting closer, my eyes are fully adjusted to the darkness now and I can see that I am only inches from the bucket. Pulling my pants down to mid thigh, I sit right down, taking the load off my legs. The weight of the bucket confirms that it is still full of water.

My legs feel better, but the pressure on my exit hole is now too much to bare, I can feel it opening and closing against my will. "Fuck you" I whisper, willing it painfully back up stream. As the conversation in the hallway reaches my door, the pain becomes too much and I let slip a little.

The room seems a little less hot as I realise that the pressure is off, but that I have about half a shit hanging out of my arse. A little push and a gentle splash later, last nights dinner slips into the mop water like a navy seal.

I breathe a quiet sigh of relief as I hear the conversation move down the hallway, followed by the eager slapping of children's feet on the tiles. Two minutes and they'll be round the corner and my little version of hell will be over.

Then I feel the vibrating of the phone in my pocket. It feels like forever as I battle with the reality, my mind begging to me, telling me that it's not happening. The fucking alarm, I think as I piece together what is coming.

"rrrrrrinnnnnnng" I knew it was coming, but in the confines of the mop cupboard, in my present state of semi nudity, the noise was like a fire alarm. "Damn my body," I think as it convulses on it's own, rocketing me up to a standing position.

As my hand jams itself into my pocket, the burnt part of my back is reintroduced to the hot water pipe. launching forward to get away, I explode out into the light of the hallway.

"Daddy, daddy!" Alexis' high pitched squeal of excitement pierces through the light. I can't see anything, but I can feel my sweaty hand reefing at my shorts, trying to get the phone out. I can imagine the look on Sharny's face, watching me roll on the floor, drowned in sweat, pants half way down my legs, stinking of shit.

Not a peep from her. "They're in shock" I think as I finally wiggle my pants up and free the phone.

"Daddy, daddy... poopoo" says Alexis as my eyes adjust to the light. Kicking the door shut, I muster a pathetic "surprise" as I turn to face the girls.

I can honestly say now that I know what it's like to escape death, because no sooner had I turned around to see the girls, did they come back around the corner. They had not seen any of the past few seconds, and confirming my brave hope, Rach comes up to me saying "what a good surprise" as she throws her arms around me.

"Daddy, poopoo" says Alexis. I can feel her little hand tapping me on the bum, bringing attention to the smell.

"Alexis must have done a poo," I mumble as I see her face wrinkle up. "I better go change it."

"Be quick," says Rach "I've got lots of presents for you guys, and I want to see your faces when you open them"

Scooping Alexis up, I mince into her room and slam the door.

"Little snitch" I giggle as I tickle the confused look off her face.

"Quick, nappy off" cleaning myself with her wipes, tears of laughter pour down my cheeks.

A few minutes later, we're on the couch, sipping on soda water to cover the giggle that keeps erupting from my lips. Rach has handed out all her presents and says to me. "I know you don't like me buying you any chocolate, so I got you a book, it's pretty lame, I'm sorry".

"Damn right it's lame" I think, tearing the wrapping paper off. Her words starting to register, I begin to feel guilty. "That's so thoughtful of you," I say. She really does know me well. For my birthday, she bought me a massive block of chocolate, which started a binge that lasted until well past christmas.

"Maybe she's not so cruel after all" I think, still buzzing from the enormous amounts of adrenalin flowing in my blood.

That night, I apologised to Sharny about Rach, and admitted that I was being silly calling her an evil witch. "I really thought she would bring chocolate again. I've only just got over my last downward spiral of food addiction from Easter, and I really didn't want her to start me off again. What did she get you?"

"Um, just some books too" she mumbled defensively, thumbing through the pages in my book.

"Oh yeah, what on?" I ask, sensing the lie.

"Nothing much."

"Nothing much?"

"I can't lie to you. She brought me a selection box of hand made Belgian chocolate"

There is an army of fat guys living inside me. It takes an enormous amount of willpower to get them under control, but once they're under control, they become petulant. Kicking at the walls of my stomach and pulling at my oesophagus if they smell any type of junk food.

It doesn't even have to be junk food. If I open a bag of oranges, I can't stop eating them until they're all gone. Then, when I'm at my weakest, the fat guys inside me seize control.

They overpower me, forcing me to drive them to the cold foods section of the supermarket. On my way home, I find myself calling the pizza shop, mouth stuffed with icecream.

What starts as an orange, ends up being a 3 week bender that easily has me packing on at least 10 kilos.

I'm addicted to food. I fight my addiction every day. Unlike drug, cigarette or alcohol addiction, food addiction is not only socially acceptable, it's available everywhere, and necessary for survival.

An alcoholic can hide from alcohol exposure, avoiding pubs, parties and bottle stores, but there is nowhere to hide from a food addiction. It's embarrassing and illegal to drink booze or take drugs in public, but food is consumed anywhere.

An alcoholic can go his whole life without ever touching another drink. You can't do that with food. If you're addicted to food like I am, you have to ride your emotions like a skilled horseman holding back a powerful stallion that just wants to gallop.

You can't keep it in the pen for a few days, because as soon as you open the gate it will bolt. You have to allow it just enough running to keep it from running away. It takes enormous amounts of energy to regain control, but I have to. The greater part on me refuses to yield to the unbearable force of my hunger. Day after day, I battle with it.

Last night, listening to the yelling and screaming of the fat guys inside, I watched the chocolates fall one by one into the sink. The boiling water guarantees that they will disappear down the drain. They've tricked me before into throwing chocolate into the bin; hours later, my guard down, I would find myself digging through the trash. I wasn't going to risk it this time.

Yesterday, I won the battle with the fat guys. Sharny must have seen my desperation and agreed to keep junk food out of the house forever, she even rang Rach and asked her to never bring chocolate for anyone.

I feel like a terrible dad. Because I have no self control, my kids have to suffer. I'm so sad I could cry, but I won't because the cleaner is here, and she's picking up toys off the floor around me so she can mop it.

Oh fuck.

Be Entrepreneurial About Your Exercise

4.30am on a Friday. Alexis was 3 days old. We had just had our first night at home with her and were preparing for our second. We had clicked up about 6 hours of sleep between us over the past 3 days and were both wandering around like ships at night, too tired for all but the most basic of human needs. Too tired to talk.

CHAAAAANGGGGGG...

The usual melodic sms chime sounded like a chainsaw, cutting deep inside my brain.

I'll be there. but i have to be gone by 5.30

Too tired to speak, my internal voice was screaming at me. I had forgotten that one of our clients, Dave, was flying in and wanted a session at 5am. We lived 15 minutes from the studio, and I hadn't showered, shaved or brushed my teeth in 3 days.

Normally, people don't notice their own stink; when I open the door to my teenager's room in the morning, it feels like I've been slapped, but he is oblivious to the stench. That day, even in my exhausted state, I could smell myself. It was offensive. But I had struggled to care until now.

When did I last eat? Have I got time for a coffee?

Stupid questions flooded my brain. A had to get clean fast, and get out to the studio. I usually come up with great workouts and ideas in the shower, but today I couldn't. *What am I going to do in 30 minutes?*

Sleep deprived decision making is pure comedy. By the time I had met Dave at the door of his taxi, 40 different ideas had entered my brain and left. I had even forgotten about the 30 minute time cap and after rehashing the birth story to Dave, I asked why his taxi was still waiting outside.

"I have to leave at 5.30. We've got 15 minutes."

The words barely registered in my brain, I was staring at the whiteboard trying to collect my thoughts when Dave's voice cut through.

"Cool, let's do it."

Apart from our books, seminars and programs, we make a living training professional athletes and high end CEO's, all of whom share extremely competitive natures. Today, this trait would change my life.

On the whiteboard, written in red was the following:

deadlift

power clean
chins
dips
3 sets of 8

It's a workout we still use today for contact sports to increase impact power. It usually takes around an hour to complete, because we work with very high weights and recovery of 2 or so minutes between sets.

Dave, CEO of a multinational company was no rugby player. Lucky for me, he was a very direct, aggressive competitive person - something he attests his success to. I had been working with him for a while now and he was getting very strong, his technique had become spot on.

We set up a bar with 60kg on it and then I witnessed something awesome.

I never asked Dave how he was, too caught up in my own self pity, but looking back now, he was livid. The taxi had picked him up from Brisbane International Airport and brought him straight here, an hour's drive.

He'd been away on a business trip to Japan, an unexpected suicide trip that would have him forced to witness his Japanese suppliers handing over their business to Dave's competitor. He stood to lose millions and millions of dollars and when he told his wife, she had asked for a divorce.

The man was angry and needed a release. Normally in these situations, we do sparring, but I didn't know. Outwardly, he seemed so at ease, but internally he was burning up.

And then he let loose.

He finished his first set of deadlifts and immediately started the power cleans, once he was finished with those he ran to the chinup bar and pumped out his chins, pausing for a brief moment before dipping.

He was moving so fast I didn't want to tell him he had it all wrong, it was meant to be 3 sets of 8 of each, but he was doing everything at once. It was madness. It was magical. In his rage, he did the whole workout unbroken in less than 5 minutes.

Lying on the floor, gasping for air was a new man. Where before, I could see the disappointment of a man who never quite succeeds burning through his eyes, there was now just joy. He was excited, he was energetic, he was euphoric. It was contagious. I could feel his energy. I could feel his pride.

When he finally peeled himself off the floor he confessed the reasons for his rage, but without malice. He was merely making an account. He talked about his wife and Japan as though they were irrelevant. He joked, laughed and looked like he was dancing. I had never seen this side of him and told him so.

"I don't know who I am right now. I haven't felt this happy since I was about 5 years old. It's weird man, but I like it, I feel young again, full of potential, and that energy and optimism I had when I first started in business... I feel that right now."

And then he was gone, the tail lights of the taxi disappeared round the corner as I stood there wondering. Excited. I was alone in this massive building, the deep bass of the music a metronome for my heart beat.

I picked up the bar to put it away and put it back down again. Then picked it up. The put it down, up, down, up, down... deadlifts, power cleans, chins and dips. 3 rounds as fast as I could. I collapsed on the ground like a wet towel.

What the fuck did I just do?

I didn't even warm up. My heart was pounding so hard in my ears that it now drowned out the music.

Like the sound of a motorbike on the highway, I could feel it coming... faint, distant. Louder and louder before it hit me. Like diving into a pool on a hot summers day, the energy engulfed me. First pleasure, then excitement, then joy. I started giggling. Giggling turned into laughter and before I knew it I was moving again.

It was like I had just drank 100 cups of coffee - I was buzzing. I was euphoric. I was too excited to entertain my disbelief. I skipped to the car and sang at the top of my voice all the way home.

The next few hours were like an awakening. It was as though all the clutter had been swiped away so I could see my path, I could see my role as a father and a husband. Something magical was happening to me. I was alive.

Poor Sharny thought I was on drugs. I danced around all day and couldn't sleep that night. By the time the next night came, the euphoria had worn off and I slept a sleep so deep and relaxing that I woke after 5 hours feeling as though I had slept for days.

I checked my phone to see the time and found a message from Dave, the man described by his family and employees as an aggressive, angry heartless man.

I love you guys

That day started a quest for understanding that has ultimately led to the writing of this book. Why did that happen?

We've been able to replicate that feeling time and time again in our own training and our clients. I tell you, it is very addictive. One of our athletes says it's like cocaine, except that it lasts way longer. We've never tried cocaine, but now we won't need to.

Time Is Immaterial, Intensity Is Essential.

Before that day, we used to believe that we would need to work out for at least 45 minutes to get any kind of result. There was no point in exercising for less than that. All gym classes are on the hour and go for an hour. When we ran, we aimed to run for an hour.

But it's not working. If you run for an hour, you spend the entire time conserving your energy.

If you are trying to get fitter, you need to promote an adaptive response. Which means that your body will adapt to the stress you give it. This is the principle behind progressive overload - bodybuilders slightly increase the weights they lift every time.

Training for fat loss and wellness for an hour forces you to think conservatively, so to survive the hour, your body will spend almost all of the hour at submaximal effort. The only possible adaption in this scenario is to go for longer, which is impractical and can put overuse stress on your joints.

In strength training, it is the rep that cannot be completed that triggers the adaptive response (getting stronger). In strength training we therefore don't train athletes for a specific time, we train them for a single, specific lift that they cannot complete.

For fitness training, we train athletes for a specific intensity that they cannot complete. If you work at an intensity that is so far removed from your body's day to day activities, your body will be forced to adapt. You will get fitter. The next time you try that intensity, you will be able to sustain it. Increase the intensity and do it again - it is the only way to get fitter.

Training for an hour at submaximal intensity puts a limit on the adaptation you can achieve. This is why so many gym class attendees complain about hitting a plateau with their weight loss or fitness. They have adapted and the body no longer needs to get fitter.

One hour sessions don't serve the gym attendee any way. They were never designed with you in mind. They are a commercial decision.

Gym owners initially didn't want people wandering around the gym aimlessly, because it looks crowded. So they created classes to get most of the people off the floor so they can sell more memberships. Gym instructors are paid on an hourly basis, so it is much easier bookkeeping to track their sessions if they are an hour long than if they are varied.

One hour sessions are designed to make the gym owners life easier, not the gym goer.

As business people we can applaud the gym owner's plan, but we can choose to use this entrepreneurial thinking for our own benefit, our own athletic gain.

Robert Kiyosaki, author of the Rich Dad series says that one of the first steps to becoming an entrepreneur is realising that rich people get paid for a result, poor people get paid by the hour. The result is important, the time is immaterial. When an entrepreneur realises this, he will never work for wages again.

As a kid, my dad would pay me for chores, like mowing the lawn. I used to hate doing it, and negotiated my dad into paying me 20 dollars to do it for him, because it would take him 2 hours and that was 10 dollars an hour.

I was not a very patient boy. Pair this with my reputation as a lazy child, I wasn't surprised when dad only agreed to pay me the 20 dollars when the job was done. Smart man.

Expecting me to give up half way, and only have half a lawn for himself to mow, he went into town with mum. I had a million better things to do than mow the lawn, but I wanted the cash. So I goofed off for an hour and a half, doing whatever it is I wanted to do, and then spent 30 minutes mowing the lawn.

I worked like a child possessed. Instead of walking with the mower, I ran. I finished the job in half an hour and earned my 20 bucks. I realised then that I would never work for an hourly rate, and have yet to do so. Working for an hourly rate means that somebody else dictates my time and my value.

Why let someone else dictate your time in the gym? Be entrepreneurial about your fitness. Do the job as fast as you can, not for as long as you can. You'll get a better result, and gain a sense of achievement too. Then you can go and spend the rest of the hour doing whatever *you* want.

The Fountain Of Youth

If you go to the gym for wellbeing, try changing your spin class or pump class for a quick, intense full body workout. When you do exercises that incorporate a lot of movement at a high speed, with a competitive spirit, your body releases two hormones, called IGF-1 and HGH. These two combined are what we call the *fountain of youth*.

Aging clinics across the world inject synthetic HGH into 60 year olds so that they can reverse the aging process. Patients report increases in vitality, injury rehabilitation, reversed arthritis, balding and osteoporosis, increased sex drive, reduced body fat, increased muscle mass, feelings of self worth and importance.

Essentially, these patients are paying huge sums of money to feel young again. High intensity full body resistance exercise (HIFBRE) [said *high fibre*] releases it for free, is completely natural and it only takes 5 -15 minutes.

Not only does this type of training make you feel good, it also curbs hunger, and changes your body's metabolism in such a way as to burn fat as a primary source of fuel for 24-36 hours after the workout.

When Sharny and I train now, it is 90% HIFBRE. It helps with so much of our lives. Our CEO clients are addicted to it too. Everyone who does this type of training does not want to go back to any other kind.

HIFBRE translates across sports and codes. Professional rugby players, tennis players, golfers, swimmers, rowers, basketball players, boxers, MMA, runners and triathletes that we have conditioned or been involved with all revolutionised their fitness from the explosive power and lightning recovery afforded by HIFBRE training.

Try it one day and tell us what you think...

Stress Adaptation

You've heard of fight or flight, right?

Fight or flight is the natural, genetic inbuilt response an animal has to stress. It is a reaction, and therefore uncontrollable. A mouse, foraging for food in the barn, hears something crack in the darkness, it's too close to figure out what it is, or if it is a danger, what does it do?

It runs away; Flight.

A snake, slithering around in the dark, hears something crack in the dark, it's too close to figure out what it is, or if it's in danger, what does it do?

It strikes; Fight.

This reaction to the stress does not even register in the consciousness of the mouse or snake until well after the event. An animal's response to stress is important, because it is a matter of life or death. Whether it is right or wrong is irrelevant, because if it is not a danger, the mouse has run from nothing, and the snake has struck at nothing, no harm done.

What is relevant in the animal kingdom is that the reaction, the response to stress, happens instantaneously. A split second delay for decision making could mean certain death. Fight or flight is unconscious, completely out of the animal's control.

Humans still have the fight or flight response.

Growing up, Julius and his brothers used to hide in doorways and behind corners to jump out and scare one another. David, the youngest one would always jump back, Daniel, the older one would lash out. David had a flight response to the stress, Daniel had a fight response.

Naturally, David would end up being Julius' victim the most, because Daniel's fight response was a little tricky when wedged into a tight corner with no exit route.

We'll let the story continue in Julius' own words:

The secret to a good scare is patience.

If you can wait long enough to catch your victim off guard, you've got a much better chance of getting an awesome response. An embarrassingly high pitched squeal is a prized trophy for a 10 year old boy, bent on scaring his brother.

One dark night, after a particularly scary movie, we all went to sleep. Except Daniel. Daniel, who still to this day has an evil addiction to frightening people, waited for over an hour behind the nearly closed toilet door for one of us to wake, bladder full, desperate to empty it.

When he heard the bed sheets rustling, he adjusted his horror mask, tightened the sheet around him and took a slow, deep breath. Filling his lungs to capacity, he steadied himself to roar at the poor fool who was about to open the door. David, this time.

Stumbling through the dark, half asleep, David opened the door.

Everybody in the house heard the roar, and probably everyone in the whole neighbourhood, it was so loud, and Daniel had put a particularly terrifying rasp in it that got the whole family running to see what had happened.

Sprinting around the corner, expecting to see Daniel rolling on the floor laughing, I was completely surprised. Daniel was lying on the floor, motionless. David was standing over him, hands balled into fists, muscles quivering like a race horse.

Looking back now, we can appreciate the magnitude of what happened. Back then, I was just disappointed that the scaring game had become too risky, both my brothers were too dangerous to scare.

That memory has stayed with Julius for years, he knew there was something important about it, but never could put his finger on it. Now he knows.

David had managed to *change his reaction*, his fight or flight response.

Fight or flight is a reaction, it is unconscious, uncontrollable. That's what we believed. Not any more. If David could control the uncontrollable, what were the possibilities for us, for our clients. For athletes.

This is a very, very interesting puzzle. How did David retrain his unconscious brain, and how could we replicate the result?

Julius and his brothers would scare one another every chance they got. For David, the scaring game happened 20 or 30 times a day, so he had a lot of exposure to the stress, and could therefore steadily retrain his subconscious mind.

Julius put this theory to test for a State Rugby Union backline he trained in 2009.

The thing about coaching rep teams compared to club teams is that you don't have to set a game plan around weaker players. In a rep team, every player has earned their spot and is good at what they do. Where coaching rep teams *is* a struggle, is that everybody is good, and can appear to be 'ball hogs'.

Under the pressure of high stakes games, such as grand finals, most representative players become ball hogs, unconsciously throwing the game plan. To the frustrated coach, understanding this is vital to success. The player may come from a club team where they are the best player, and therefore *the* game plan. Used to being given the ball under pressure, he is expected to work his magic.

In high level team sport though, the opponent's players are as good, if not better than your players. And in rugby, the combination of ball hog and good opposition defence means that your player will be isolated and subsequently lose possession of the ball.

Many times we have seen coaches storming the sidelines, yelling at their players, pulling their own hair out in frustration, and it is *always* about the same thing. "He doesn't listen to me! No matter how much we practice, he just does what he wants!"

Armed with my understanding of stress response, I decided then to analyse this phenomenon. Contrary to what the coach says, the players are not prima donnas, they do not even like what they have done. It is an unconscious behaviour, which all high stakes, high pressure sport becomes.

So instead of telling the players what was wrong with them, compounding the problem by crushing their confidence, we set about retraining their reaction under stress.

In most team sports, the difference between a good team and an excellent team is their ability to execute strategic movements. In rugby, it is the backline whose job it is to run in different directions, a beautiful dance, designed to confuse the defence, thus opening a hole for a player to run through and score.

These back line moves are practiced over and over and over again until they can be done with eyes closed. Where it falls apart is translating that practice to game time. A really good defensive team will put pressure on the backline by rushing them, forcing errors.

So, what would happen then, if we could practice these moves under enormous amounts of manufactured pressure?

In rugby, the distance between back line and the defence is generally 10 metres. So in training, we cut it down to 9 metres. Then 8, then 7, right down to 1 metre - something that would never happen. Much to the disgust of the other coaches, we appeared to be practicing something unrealistic.

Once the players became comfortable with reducing the decision making time, we added unpredictability. Defenders coming from all angles, in front, behind and the side - once again, something that would not happen in a real game.

We practiced moves where one player would at the last second not join the move, or get 6 defensive players to rush a single man.

Over time, the players became comfortable with this enormous, unpredictable pressure we had manufactured, and appeared to think, and make game winning decisions incomprehensibly fast.

Come tournament time, the backline moves were no longer one dimensional, they were fluid, able to change while they were being executed. That team, much smaller than the competition and having come last the year before, went through the tournament unbeaten.

They were able to score from any part of the field, because the stress adaptation was complete. We had retrained the athletes reactions, we had retrained their unconscious minds. We had controlled the uncontrollable.

The profoundness of what we had discovered became evidently clear by the shocked looks on the player's faces when scoring - they were playing unconsciously, and *didn't even know how they were doing it*, they just did it.

As an athlete, you can reprogram your stress response. But what does this mean for mum or dad, or business executive whose stresses are not visible, stresses that may build up and be stacked on top of one another.

Most modern day human stresses cannot be reacted upon with a fight or flight response. They get bottled up, and like a pressure chamber, pushing on our walls, waiting for a weakness, waiting for a release.

Often stress builds up and multiplies so fast we just have no time to release it. It is scary too, when a man finally blows his top, no longer able to hold the stress in, he acts unconsciously, uncontrollably. If his reaction is unfavourable, something we might not even expect, it is too late to change after the event. People are hurt, the damage has been done.

High intensity exercise mimics high stress. You can reprogram yourself and your reaction or capacity for stress through high intensity exercise. Problems you may face in your life should be expressed in your exercise.

Rather than hiding from your animal instincts, you can be open to them, allow them to take control, then observe them and retrain them if necessary. This way, you can control the uncontrollable.

Be An Explorer

Who was more successful; Nostradamus, the great adventurer, or Alexander, the great conquerer?

Scholars studying the life of Alexander will tell you that he was a deeply depressed man. It seems that conquering the known world never afforded him any true happiness, only bitterness.

Nostradamus, on the other hand, was a joyous soul. The great explorer's life, although punctured by great sadness, loss and disaster, was underpinned by happiness.

Nostradamus and Alexander. Both held the world in their hands, one drew happiness from it, the other was haunted by it.

Why?

Why is it that kids are always laughing, but adults seldom do? Why is it that a drunk laughs more than a sober man?

The happiest adult I know is a lady called Carren Smith. Carren's life story reads like a Shakespearian tragedy. After her fiance committed suicide, she went to Bali with her two best friends to cheer up. While there she survived the Bali bombing only to wake up to the news her best friends had both died, and she had a partially crushed skull. She has always wanted children, is amazing with children, but has had her ovaries removed. Carren has every right to be depressed... She is not.

The most depressed person I know is a man called Damien Franklin [*name changed for privacy*]. To the outside world, Damien is the epitome of success. He is wealthy beyond our wildest dreams, he has a stunning wife who loves him dearly, 3 kids who are high achievers and a career that sees him pressing flesh with the most influential people on earth. Damien makes a living practicing an art he loves, he is good at. Damien *hates* his life.

Why?

Damien approaches every single day with purpose. His life is lived on purpose. He is what all the self help success books want you to become. He is the embodiment of single minded purpose.

Carren is not.

She is also very successful, but where she is different to Damien is that her tragedies have afforded her a completely different view of her life. Carren has lived in her nightmares, she has allowed them in, she has let them take her.

Why does this make her happy, while Damien remains sad?

I'll tell you soon, but first, a story about Carren.

When Carren first came to us for fitness coaching, she described how burpees made her pass out. It had something to do with the piece of building that had been lodged in her skull in Bali 10 years ago. She said that we shouldn't be alarmed, just forewarned. It happened a fair bit.

As part of our initial assessment of athletes, we test dexterity, core stability and pelvic alignment through a simple one legged toe touch. I asked Carren to try it. When she came back up from her first one, I noticed her eyes glazing over. I asked if she was OK, and she said she needed to lie down for a bit.

I stopped the session instantly and proceeded with a stretch and massage. The stretch happens on the floor, but the massage on a bench. Carren was sitting in front of me as I worked my hands up and down her back, rubbing and prodding, learning about the nuances of my new athletes posterior chain.

I was firing questions at her to test her alertness and concentration span, when I noticed she stopped answering. I carried on the massage in silence, thinking she was sick of my babbling, when she said once again "I need to lie down"

I really, really wanted to understand the process she went through with a faint, so that I could know her limits, I needed to know the signs so that I was able to pull back. I asked her what she felt, immediately before she passes out.

"I feel so hot inside my body, then my eyes start to get pins and needles; then I know that the blackness is coming."

"Have you ever tried to fight it?" I asked

She had a very stern look on her face, so I quickly followed with "you know, when you hear stories of people nearly dying, they can see death coming, and just turn the other way, they fight it. Same with sleep, sometimes you can feel sleep coming, and you can turn the other way and fight it, have you ever tried to turn the other way when you start to feel the pins and needles?"

I then remembered that she had in fact nearly died, so asked her what that was like. Had she fought off death, had she turned the other way when she saw the bright white light?

"No, there was never even a thought of death, I never even let it register. It wasn't planned or on purpose, thinking back though, I know now that I just didn't have any belief whatsoever that this was the end."

"And no, I haven't tried fighting it, I just accept it and let go". I could see she was internalising - she was talking more to herself than to me, she was analysing herself.

Carren is an amazing woman, apart from being very joyful and inspiring to be around, she is a very well respected and loved thought leader - a modern day prophet if you will, so it wasn't a surprise when she agreed to try fighting it.

"Right now?"

"Why not?" she said. Her eyes looking internally, not really focussing on me, but scanning, scanning like a giant computer - exploring the possibilities.

"Are you sure you want to do this, I don't want you to do anything against your will, so it is totally your call."

"I want to do it, I just know that if I faint I will vomit, and I don't like to vomit"

"Let's go outside onto the lawn then" I promised her that I'd catch her. But not her vomit.

She agreed.

When I was a kid, we used to make each other faint by holding our heads between our knees, then standing up really fast. This was my 'highly advanced technique' for getting her to faint.

She held her head in between her knees. Eons passed as I whispered to her - "refuse it, just fight it away, it is not happening to you"

Everything seemed to come closer, the birds looked brighter. I could even hear the whirr of the neighbours dishwasher. Time seemed to stand still. Something special was about to happen. something... profound.

"Stand up fast" I command. And she does.

I hold her arms gently but firmly. If she spews, it's going all over me, but I don't care because I am *not* letting her fall. I'm staring straight into her eyes, watching, waiting to see the darkness, the blankness.

"Nothing" she says.

"Are you sure?"

"Nothing," she shakes her head "not even the spew feeling, nothing. no blackness, no pins and needles, nothing. I feel so tall."

"I feel so tall" she repeats, convincing herself that it's true. The giant computer scanning, scanning. Her internal dialogue going into overdrive, the guru's self analysis had begun.

I knew something special had happened, and I'm sure that by the time this book has been published this story will form one of the parables in her amazing teachings, but for us it highlighted something very important.

If Carren hadn't tried to faint, she would never have known that she could fight it. Why did she try to faint? It's the exact reason she is happy and Damien is not. It is the same reason that Nostradamus was joyful, but Alexander depressed, it is why children laugh and adults don't.

Carren, like the child, is an adventurer in her own life. Carren approaches her life with a sense of discovery, where Damien approaches his with purpose.

Damien's life is one of achievement, his purpose is to become rich. But what is rich? There is no definition. Every time Damien reaches what he thought previously was his rich level, he sees that it is not enough. Damien is chasing an unachievable goal, and in the meantime missing the real adventure and joy in his life.

Carren, Nostradamus and children don't focus on their long term goals. They focus on right now. Right here and right now. They don't hold anything back for later, because for all they know, later never comes.

Tragedy has struck Carren for absolutely no reason. You can't put brain damage in your 10 year plan! Carren sees every day as an adventure, her only purpose is to discover.

In the last chapter we talked about exercise as a metaphor for life. If you want to really understand yourself, approach every workout as an adventure. Don't save anything for later, don't stop at exhaustion, because just beyond your comfort zone is where the magic happens. Like Carren would say "you deserve to know yourself".

What maketh the man (or woman)?

Every now and then, when we're feeling a little detached, we will approach a workout with a different mindset. A completely different mindset. To do this takes a lot of mental preparation and a very good training buddy or coach. It's best to do this with someone who knows you well, knows your current limits.

It can be any workout, but remember that time is a substitute for intensity. So if you don't have much time, you have to work at extremely high intensity. If intensity is not your thing, then go for time. One of the best exercises for this is running.

If we have time, we'll just keep running for as far as we can. Sometimes hours, sometimes days. The faster we run, the sooner it happens. There comes a point, long after 'hitting the wall' where we have tapped further into our energy stores than we ever have before.

When we feel like we can't run anymore, tears streaming down our faces, muscles aching right through to the bone, the workout begins. The discovery begins. The mindset changes. We go down the rabbit hole. We swallow the adventure pill.

Try it.

Internalise, look at yourself from above, analytically. Observe what your body is doing, observe how it is reacting. Feel how it is trying to pull your consciousness back to the pain. Don't let it. Just drift. Explore, discover. See what's there. What's beyond that frontier you are afraid of.

Does pain go away, does it get worse, how much can you actually take?

How far will your body go without your consciousness there to pull on the reigns?

If you don't have time, just run faster. We find ultra distance running takes longer to reach, but the drift, the euphoria, the discovery lasts longer, but if you run at an 800m pace for 5, maybe 10 km, you'll get there sooner. Sometimes much sooner.

You'll know it when you're there - you'll hurt more and more and more. Everything in you will tell you to slow down. But you won't because you know that if you slow down you'll miss it. Like an aeroplane taking off, you just have to go faster.

Your feet will hurt, your lungs will burn, you may even begin to cry. You'll know then, that you are close. Keep going, faster. Faster. Faster.

And then like magic, it happens. Absolute serenity. You take off. You're flying. You're at peace.

You'll see everything about yourself in crystal clarity for those brief moments. Clutch onto them, because like a delicious dream, you know you're going to wake up soon. Hold on as long as you can, explore. Discover.

Like Carren Smith, like Nostradamus - right here, right now; you're an explorer.

Understanding Tall Poppy Syndrome

Something in our human DNA powers the need for improvement. From when we're born, we're striving for an always changing goal. As we write this, Danté our son is just about to start walking.

We never taught him how. He just learned to pull himself into a standing position against a wall or a box, or shelf. Every waking moment, he would work at it. Steely determination in his eyes, frustration in his little voice, until he got up on his two wobbly little legs. He'd yell a warcry of triumph before his knees would buckle and he would come crashing down with a thump.

Poor little fella, every time he fell he would burst into tears, but nothing we could do could console him, if we picked him up, he'd cry until we put him back down. As soon as he was down, he'd crawl to the wall where he would begin the painful, slow process of climbing again.

Alexis, only a year older, and much better on her feet thought she was very helpful. She'd wait until he was up, and then help him back down to earth with a push on his chest. Thump.

Tears streaming from his face, bottom lip poked out, he'd immediately roll over and crawl back for the wall. Not a moment's rest, not even a pause; thump, roll, crawl, climb.

As adults, we're no different. The process is the same... thump, roll, crawl, climb... Except that some of us focus more on the thump. We allow it to define us. Victim mentality, some call it. The baby cheers when he stands up, the victim cheers when he falls down. "Look at me" he cries, "I'm suffering adversity..."

You can only fall, if you have climbed. You can only cry once for each climb. The victim becomes a loser when he allows failure to define him. He stops climbing, choosing to instead lie on the ground saying "I keep falling, I keep falling".

When the leader falls, he states the truth; "I have fallen."

What makes the difference?

To be the leader is to have suffered the victim mindset for long enough that you realise nobody cares. The leader then stops complaining, and begins climbing.

There is nothing wrong with the victim mindset, it is a part of learning - great lessons are learnt when we fall hard enough and often enough that we get emotional. Every innocent little child has said, tears streaming down their face "I'll never get to [ride the bike/ climb the rope/talk to the sweetheart...]

But they do.

It is not natural to pause too long between thump and roll To stay in the victim seat after the lesson has been learnt is dangerous. Once we have kicked and screamed and had our little hissy fit, we *must* get back up. If we do not, if we choose to stay there for a little longer, we start to look around. And when we look around, we never like what we see.

When a child looks around for the first time, they meet their lifelong enemy. As soon as he looks into those beady eyes, the child is bound. A painful bind that lasts forever. From that moment on, the centipede buries himself into the child, wrapping around him, tightening the grip with every breath. The centipede has a charming smile and bright eyes, and whispers gently "everything will be OK, I'm here to protect you..."

Listen quietly for a second. Do you hear that voice inside your head? Everybody has one, the voice inside your head that protects you, whispers to you all day. Can you hear him now, what's he saying?

Like a politician, he is very cunning, and very convincing. And just like a politician, he appears to be helping you, but really he is just trying to keep his job - he wants to remain in power.

Rugby World Cup, 2011. New Zealand born Quade Cooper, undoubtedly the greatest talent in world rugby at the time, is playing for the Australian wallabies. If anyone is going to upset the favourites, it is Quade Cooper. Only weeks before the start of the tournament, he spear headed one of the greatest upsets in Tri Nations history, bringing the great All Blacks to their knees with an understrength, youthful Wallabies team.

Quade Cooper is going to his birth country, his family, his blood to have his crack at winning the Webb Ellis Cup. Do they greet him with open arms? Do they love that this amazing talent was born of their soil?

No, they absolutely slam him. He is branded public enemy number 1. In the streets, he is abused by locals, he is called a traitor. He is spat at, and threatened. Every game he plays, the homeland crowd boos him. Every time he comes close to the sideline, he can hear the hate.

His confidence begins to take a toll, and so does his gameplay. By the third game, it is obvious that he is not coming back. We give massive credit to his coach, Robbie Deans for believing in him, but the voice of one man can not drown out the shouts of a nation. Cooper never recovers, and his team suffers.

London Olympics 2012, hot favourites to win the men's 4x100m swimming relay is Australia, dubbed the 'giant killers', and led by the fastest swimmer on earth, 21 year old James, the Missile Magnussen.

In an interview before the race, the Missile confidently states that he never gets nervous, the giant killers will win.

The race comes and the Missile misfires, Australia come 4th. Favourites to win gold, they don't even finish on the podium. The media smells blood, the public want answers. In the interview immediately after the race, Magnussen is distraught "I don't know what to say" he mumbles, pulling back behind his teammates, embarrassed and ashamed.

For the next few days, nothing but outright hate is plastered on the social networks. "How dare he hide behind his teammates, the arrogant prick" the media use him for headline fodder, he is the embarrassment of the nation. He has let his country down.

Cooper and Magnussen are confidence athletes, born leaders. They perform best when they eliminate pressure, and compete with supreme confidence. So what went wrong?

It is the same in both situations, and it is the same reason you and I find it hard to get fit, or lose weight, or become rich.

4 years in the making, it has come down to this. We mortals, have deadlines that come and go. These guys' deadlines are 4 years apart. They work more hours than we ever have, for less pay than we do, for a goal so far into the future, we can only pretend to understand. For many, there is only this one chance. 4 years is the maximum life span of many athletes.

James and Quade have done all they can, and are hoping that it is enough. Read now with empathy as we take you deep into the psyche of the athlete...

In his mind, he will retrace the last 4 years. The magnitude of the task ahead of him is so thick, he can feel it. He can taste it. He'll be scanning his body for any sign of weakness, any twinge, any doubt.

The butterflies in his stomach will not settle, and his backside is raw from so many nervous trips to the toilet. He is not hungry and feels sick at the thought of food. He drinks water mechanically. He can't think about anything else other than how slow time is going.

As the seconds tick by, he will internalise. His nervous conversations seem to happen outside of him. they don't register – like people talking in the hallway. He's surrounded by thousands of people, but is all alone.

Except for the voice inside his head, the centipede.

Swimmers know this voice well. They spend hours upon hours with it – they can not escape it. They must embrace it.

Under pressure, the voice is a cold heartless bastard. An athlete's internal voice doesn't want him to get hurt, so it will come up with convenient reasons as to why he will fail. It will present them quickly, one after the other in a very, very convincing fashion.

The only combat an athlete has for this, is his confidence. A very strong, convincing internal voice, needs a very strong, convincing external voice.

The reporters and interviewers may think it has something to do with them, or that the athlete is arrogant? They flatter themselves. His answers to interviews are autonomous. He is hearing them, but only through the translation of the malicious internal voice. The voice that keeps telling him "you're going to let everyone down". The voice that keeps looking for reasons, for justification.

No athlete wants to let anyone down, so they fake confidence. It's worked before. They just have to believe it. The more they fake confidence, the quieter the inside voice. In high pressure situations, the voice is even louder. If you're the favourite, you have to shout out your confidence, just to keep sane. This is why everybody prefers to be the underdog.

Mr reporter doesn't know that. Sitting safely behind their computer, typing their nasty words. Convincing their readers that one of their own countrymen has let them down.

They have no idea how much damage their words can do. They say he will live to regret this for the rest of his life? They're right. Because when they've long gone onto their next victim, a great athlete will still be living with those cutting words.

His internal voice will be reading them to him. Again, and again. The reporter has done a great job of wounding his confidence, the only weapon he has against his internal voice.

I say headline hunting reporters are letting their countrymen down. They don't have the right to judge an athlete's effort. He's sacrificed more in the last four years for his country than the reporter's entire genetic history has.

Why is it that people hate confidence so much? Would they have preferred that he talk himself down before the event? Sacrilege. For a confidence athlete like Magnussen or Cooper, if you see modesty, be afraid for him. For that man is losing a battle with his inner voice.

Maybe we would have more medals if our critics could help our athletes, rather than find fault. When next you see an athlete showing confidence, help him out. Outward confidence is inward turmoil.

Instead of feeding his internal voice, his doubt; give fire to his confidence.

Here are some words that will go a long way to helping your athlete, and therefore your country:

"I believe in you"

We all have that internal voice, and the world sporting stage highlights it perfectly, don't think you are not immune, for when you start to stand out, others will give power to your inner voice, the centipede will whisper and you will want to listen to his convincing words.

Understand this: Unanimously, the centipede is afraid of speed, the faster you climb, the louder he'll scream, but if you do it fast enough, the wind will drown out his screams, and the chatter of others.

If you want to achieve something great, put some distance between you and the rest of the world... maybe starting with the people closest to you... the ones with the beady eyes... The ones who think they are helping you by protecting you from your dreams.

If You're Not Getting Healthy, You're Dying

18th Century Irish political philosopher Edmund Burke, often regarded as the father of modern civilisation famously declared "All that is necessary for evil to triumph is for good men to do nothing"

This means that the environment into which we are born is evil. The world will fall into chaos and pain, unless someone, hopefully a good man, does something proactive to stop this.

Maybe we know this as a child, it's innate.

Do you wonder why we are afraid of the dark?

In the absence of light, there is dark. Light is not the absence of darkness. Light is light. Dark is the absence of light. Not the opposite, rather the lack of.

Is evil then, the absence of good? Are humans evil creatures as a whole?

We don't think so. We've never met a baby who was pure evil. And even if there were such a creature, it would be a massive minority, a pinprick in the ocean of humanity. So we believe that people are good.

Circumstances are what make people evil. Julius' mother had a friend who was a police officer in the toughest part of Johannesburg, South Africa called Hillbrow - well known as one of the most dangerous places on earth.

There are hundreds of multi storey apartment buildings there that in any other city on earth would pull a large income for the owner. In Hillbrow, these buildings have been taken over by huge Nigerian crime gangs, the owners make no money.

The buildings cannot be rented. They cannot be sold. Owners cannot enter their own buildings for risk of death. Kobus van Rooyen [*name changed for privacy*] was the Hillbrow constable for years before his murder. A day in Kobus's life would haunt the toughest Australian coppa, but did Kobus think these people were evil?

No, Kobus held firm the belief that crime was circumstantial. A criminal is a victim of circumstance.

Imagine if you had lost your wallet, and were stuck in the city. An emergency at home meant that you needed to get home to see your family as fast as possible, but you just had no money *on you right now*, you were absolutely desperate.

You beg everyone on the street to help you out, but nobody does, you're crying with frustration and guilt and are praying to your god for a miracle when a car pulls up in front of you, the owner gets out in a hurry, leaving the car unlocked. You can see very clearly a $2 coin on the passenger seat of his car.

Coming up the street is a bus, with your suburb written on the front of it. You have no money for the bus, and you know the buses in the part of town don't give any charity.

He's never going to know that it's gone, he probably doesn't even know it's there. Do you take it, knowing that it will get you home on a bus? Do you reach into his car and take the $2?

If you did, you'd be committing a crime. You could go to jail for that. In some countries of the world, you could be executed. For the guy in the car, the moral is that temptation is sometimes the only motive.

While we agree with Kobus that people are generally good, we believe that greed is the motivating factor behind crime. We define crime as doing something that affects the wellbeing of another. If you steal from someone, you're affecting their wellbeing, and are therefore committing a crime.

If you poison someone, you affect their wellbeing, and are therefore committing a crime. Even if you don't know that you are committing the crime? I think that greed has a lot to answer for.

Tobacco industry - built on greed, fuelled by greed. Smoking companies even know that their product is killing their customers, but they have to feed their own children. They have to survive, so their greed (or need) preys on the greed of the consumer.

If the consumer is not thinking about their own life, if they don't have a plan for it; the bright, exciting marketing of cigarette companies will suck them in, take their money and kill them.

But it's easy to point the finger at tobacco. It was only a few years ago that smoking was prescribed to patients for a myriad of illnesses, imagined and real. Everyone believed that it was good. It was a cure. The question we should be asking is, "what cure today, is tomorrow's killer?"

Asbestos was pretty amazing… not any more. Now, there is a lot of research proving that grains, widely thought to be the base of the food pyramid are now actually responsible for a staggering number of diseases!

What about our pharmaceutical industry? Pills have side effects, but the authorities approve them based on immediacy. Not long term side effects. What about things like energy drinks, what about preservatives, colours, flavours and other food additives.

We won't know the long term effects of these chemicals for years.

In this world, there is no longer a healthy status quo. You're either getting healthy, or you're dying. The only thing needed for the triumph of evil, is for you to do nothing. Sickness and death are the default, you have to proactively work at staying healthy.

If you go to a shop with no plan for buying, you are at the mercy of the shop owner's system for selling. Buying a car or computer is a great example. If you don't go into the shop determined to buy just the computer, you'll also end up paying for a box of things you'll never use; the extended warranty, a printer and some spare cartridges.

This translates perfectly to your body, your wellbeing. If you don't have a plan for your body (your internal and external environment), you're at the mercy of someone else's plan for your body. And we can tell you categorically, nobody else cares about you. They only care about themselves.

In this world of the faceless crowd, if they can get a dollar out of you, even if they kill you for it, as long as they don't know you, even the best of people will do it. So take control of your life, your fitness, your health, your family and your finances. If you don't, someone else will.

Four Fallacies

As kids we were terrified of being caught swearing at school.

It was always fun to push the boundaries around the teachers though, yelling out words that sound like swearwords, for example "fudge!" or "ship!" One really clever kid used to say, with a perfectly timed pause, guaranteed to get teacher attention "fu'cryin' out loud!"

Kids love the word 'fallacy' because it sounds like 'phallus'. 'Phallus' means in the shape of a penis. 'Fallacy' means a myth that has been proven wrong.

"One phallus, two fallacies," the kids point at one another and laugh.

Let's expose some ugly fallacies.

Fallacy Number 1:
You Must Lose Weight *Slowly*

"I'm not on a diet, it's a way of life."

Losing weight is a transient phase. It's the transition from fat to healthy. Don't make losing weight the lifestyle. It's like taking a bus from town to the beach, declaring "I'm not going to the beach, the bus is my new way of life".

Wouldn't you rather get to the beach as fast as you possibly can?

What's the fastest way to lose weight? Starvation, fasting. It's normal, it's not dangerous. "But if I starve myself, I'll lose the muscle." This is the excuse we used to use, while sipping on a diet cola, made with enough chemicals to kill a family of penguins.

Here's something to ponder. All that fat on your body, what is it there for?

It is your fuel. It is your packed lunch. Your body isn't dumb, it will burn the fuel first, not the muscle.

While unemployed, would you kill and eat your children, rather than live off your savings?

Losing weight is like paying off debt. You're much better off paying your debt as fast as you possibly can, so you can go on living your life.

If someone is fat, and wants to be fit; and the only thing standing in their way is their fat, then wouldn't it make sense to do whatever it takes to lose it as fast as they can?

The person will then only have to lose the weight once ever. Losing weight is not meant to be a lifestyle, being obese or being fit are lifestyles, transition from the one you hate to the one you want as fast as you can.

Then, like taking a helicopter to the beach, you can enjoy the lifestyle of being fit, while all the other suckers are sitting in the bus, wondering whether it's the right bus, or wondering if the bus is going too fast, or wondering if they should just get off for a little bit because they are sick of the bus.

Lose the excess weight as fast as you can.

Fallacy Number 2:
Throw Away The Scales

As part of a Personal Training course, graduates are taught to tell their clients to "throw away the scales, because when you embark on a fitness regime, you build muscle while burning fat, so weighing yourself will give you a false sense of failure. Just go by how you feel."

This works really well for the bulk of the industry who are giving body building style programs to every one of their clients. Body building programs do exactly that: build bodies. Unfortunately due to the metabolic pathways in the body, bodybuilding programs don't burn much fat at all. In fact, they make you hungrier because you need 'muscle fuel'.

Not many Personal Trainers know this, but it suits them, because there is no accountability; the client can be strung along for months, losing no weight, because they should just go by 'how they feel'.

A man, deep in debt and desperate to get out of it goes to a bank manager for help, the bank manager, after taking his final dollars off him says "throw your bank statements away, just go by how you feel."

If the man wants to reduce his debt, he needs to look at the statements every week to see how he is going.

If you want to lose weight, then you should weigh yourself regularly and keep a tally. A score card. If the weight is not dropping, then something needs to change. The scales don't lie. If you're 2kg heavier in a week, you need to go back through your week and figure out why.

The best time to weigh yourself is as soon as you wake up, after your morning pee. If you weigh yourself at the same time every day, you mitigate the risk of having more water or more food in your belly. Because yes, your weight does fluctuate during the day.

The most important thing about weighing yourself every day is your mindset. You must avoid getting into an emotional response when you climb on the scale. Too many people get on the scale, see they have lost no weight and spend the rest of the day abusing themselves. The purpose of the weigh-in is analysis.

If a *sharnyandjulius* athlete gets on the scale and finds a higher reading, they just retrace their steps from yesterday, to find out what the cause is, so they can change it today.

Don't throw the scales away.

Fallacy Number 3:
Weight Loss Powders

Weight loss powders are unnecessary, and more than likely detrimental to your health and weight loss goals. These products prey on the desperation of obese, lazy people who lack the willpower to give up their junk food addiction.

Let's look at it logically; we'll eliminate the clever marketing (rip off the colourful label) so we can uncover one of the greatest scams on earth.

We all know that the major contributing factor to weight loss is burning more fuel than you eat. There are other factors, but they are all accelerators or decelerators. Any nutrition expert will agree that calories in less than calories out is the best place to *start*.

Simply put, look at everything you ate yesterday (imagine putting it all on the table in a pile), now take some away and just eat what's left. Logical, right?

People have somehow got themselves convinced that the best way to burn fat, is to add something to their diet because it says *burn fat* on it. That's like an unemployed man, with unsustainable credit card debt, walking into a casino and putting his rent money into a slot machine, because the sign above it says *Win $10,000*.

When it comes to any athletic problem, the first thing *we* look at is the athlete's nutrition. The athlete's question is always "what should I take?" A far more important question is "what should I take away?"

And when we say athlete, we mean anybody who is doing something physical with a goal in mind. A mum who's goal is fat loss is exactly the same as a professional sports person who's goal is more speed.

Find out what's holding you back first, otherwise you just accelerate the problem.

To put it bluntly, it's what you have been eating that's caused you to get fat, not what you haven't been eating.

What about the person who uses them to curb hunger?

Once you're full, you're no longer hungry. Full is therefore the opposite of hunger. So to curb your hunger, you need to feel full. We're all pretty good at feeling full, but our problem is that we can't stay full for long enough. The problem is therefore time.

So we need to find something that makes us feel full for longer. This means we need to find something that takes a long time to digest. Something solid would therefore take longer to digest than a liquid?

How on earth then have people managed to convince themselves that drinking something can keep them full for longer than eating something.

We don't even need to get into the ingredients list, and how you're paying way too much for a cheaply broken down version of cottage cheese, pumped full of enough heavy metals to be visibly separated with a magnet. The sugar content is high enough to cause a catastrophic insulin spike (which is felt as endless hunger), and the ingredient they use to make you feel full looks very much like a trans fat.

Trans fats (very bad fats) and unsaturated fats (good fats) can both be triglycerides. It's just that one (trans fat) is made artificially and is very sinister. In these products, triglycerides are listed separately in the ingredients list to fat. If the triglycerides were unsaturated fats (good fats), wouldn't you think the company would be telling you, proudly.

But they've called them triglycerides...interesting.

The only reason to be having a meal replacement shake is convenience. If the options are fast food, or a meal replacement shake, well - this would be a better option. Unless there isn't a supermarket or grocer close by.

Healthy eating is very simple. Eat real, unprocessed foods not chemicals. Meat, veggies, fruit, nuts and seeds. The beauty of this is you can eat as much as you want with no guilt.

The worst food you can eat is marketing.

Fallacy Number 4:
Cheat Meals

Are cigarette, alcohol or drug addicts allowed cheat days? Imagine that...

"Thankyou Miss Lohan and welcome to the Pine Rivers drug rehabilitation centre. If you just follow me, I'll take you to your room and explain how the program works.

Six days per week, you're not allowed any drugs, cigarettes or alcohol. We call these 'drug free days'. On the 7th day, called your 'cheat day', you can have all the drugs you want!

You're free to choose any day to be your cheat day, but we recommend a weekend, because you won't be busy and can therefore spend all day getting high!

It will be hard at first and you will have some bizarre cravings; speed, cocaine, heroin, whatever they are, we suggest you write them down so that on cheat day, you can take them all!

Make sure that during the week, you write your cravings down, you wouldn't want to start day one again with regret, because you forgot that last week you craved the old toot on the crack pipe now, would you?

Here's your room Ms Lohan, on the wall you'll find pictures of other people who have graduated from this course. See there, we have Mr

Sheen, and over there, we have Mr Belushi, underneath him, we have Mr Cobain and Ms Winehouse."

Cheat days. Yeah right.

Exercise Gives Energy

When it comes to food, take away before you add. What about exercise?

Exercising costs energy and time, right?

Let's see.

Kerry Pacific [*name changed for privacy*] has a magnetic personality. A mum of 2 gorgeous young girls, and a life dedicated to charity, she comes across as who she is. Generous. Kerry's kids love her, her friends love her and we love her.

Kerry and her husband are rich. The two of them started buying decrepit apartment buildings when they were younger, investing all of their income and much of their 30's into creating a successful business.

About 5 years ago, around the time her first daughter was born, the company had become so big that they were able to list it on the ASX, making them multi millionaires over night.

Shortly afterwards, eager Swiss investors saw the potential in the business and bought out all the shares on the stock market, then all the remaining shares, still owned by Kerry and her husband, taking them from rich to super rich.

Kerry is the envy of all who know her, she has 2 beautiful, well behaved girls who love her dearly. She has tons of spare time, spending most of it playing with her girls or throwing massive parties in her hilltop mansion, an architectural masterpiece overlooking the ocean and the hinterland.

Kerry's husband James absolutely adores her, and why wouldn't he? She is beautiful, happy and so much fun, and to top it off she has the body of a dancer. Approaching her 40s, but looking like a late 20's supermodel, Kerry belongs on the cover of a glamour magazine.

While Kerry's life seems magical and perfect now, it hasn't always been that way.

There was a time when she would not see her husband for months, he would be working in Singapore, and she in the back blocks of Melbourne. Money was tight, the little that they did have was invested directly back into the business.

Kerry felt trapped. She worked 16 hour a day, 7 day a week in a business that took all her money and all her time.

Early one morning, exhausted after spending hours cleaning apartments, she got a phone call from her best friend Jenny. Jenny had just bought a new super king sized bed and while her fiance was putting it together, thought she'd call Kerry and brag. Poor Kerry was sitting on her rolled up swag, back to the wall, looking at her tired, drawn out face in the bathroom mirror.

I'm wrecked, she thought. *I'm absolutely wrecked. I haven't seen my husband in months, I haven't had a day off in over 2 years, and I can't remember the last time I was outside. My friends are living the high life, buying beautiful furniture for their apartments, going to restaurants and taking luxurious, fun filled weekend getaways with each other."* Hanging up the phone before she burst into tears, Kerry pulled herself off the floor, desperate to just get out of there.

Silently weeping, she wandered aimlessly through the hallways. *There's not enough time... there's not enough time* her mind mumbled like a metronome.

Head filled with thoughts of defeat, she found herself standing in the resident's gym. On her left stood a large contraption with pin weights, seats jutting out from all angles and handles hanging from everywhere. To the right was the sauna and in front of her was the rowing machine, a tattered piece of paper sticky taped to the seat, *out of order* barely legible on the faded page.

Just another job for me, she thought, thumbing the loose foot straps. Fingers working by themselves, she set about fixing the rower as her mind wandered off.

When she came back from her daydream, she felt a new found energy. Apparently the rower was fixed and tested. She looked through her sweaty brow at the computer and noticed she had just done 5km.

"Weird", she puffed, "I don't even remember rowing. But I do remember how clearly I was thinking." On the way back to her room, she noticed he feet. They were skipping. In the shower, she started singing. *I've never sung* she thought to herself.

The day of wall scrubbing that was meant to last forever, went by in a moment. Looking at the sun set through the hallway windows, she wondered at how she could still be feeling so energetic. So *alive*. How too, had she managed to get 16 hours of work done before sunset?

The next morning, she woke up refreshed. Her sleep had been deep and restorative. Sitting up, she looked at the familiar face in the mirror and said to herself "I look younger".

Humming to herself optimistically as she ambled down the hallway she thought to herself *I must tell James*. Finding herself once again sitting on the rower, she knew her life would turn out alright. Tightening the straps, she knew what she would say to James when she saw him next.

"We're investors James, in the same way we invest our time and our money into these buildings so that they give us some back, I am investing time into exercise. Exercise is not time spent. It is time invested."

From that day on, Kerry saw her life differently. While her friends were *spending* their time and their money, she was *investing* it. While they were getting further and further into debt, she was getting out of it.

While they were getting fatter and fatter, she was getting fitter. While they were working more and more, she was becoming more efficient. While they were complaining that their husbands were spending too little time at home, she was investing what little time she had with her husband into bettering their relationship.

Nowadays, Kerry's life is easier. But does she sit back and relax? No. She invests her spare time into helping a local charity.

Her daughters love her because she invests in quality time with them, she doesn't just spend time with them. She has a deep, meaningful connection with her husband because they invest in their relationship. She looks like a supermodel mum because she invests time into her beauty. She is wealthy because she continues to invest the money she has.

And she has the energy to do it all because she invests a little bit of time every day, to exercise.

Distinguish Want From Need

Read this story:

Tuesday afternoon, the initial hum drum and excitement of school pick up and "what happened at school today" is finished. The house quietens a little as Josh sits down at the kitchen table to do his homework. Sharny wants to call Emma, but she needs to ring Jodie. As she's tiptoeing down the hallway, Josh notices her leaving and says:

"I need $5 for school tomorrow"

By the time she's finished talking to him, she only has time for one phone call. Who does she call?

Now read this story:

Tuesday afternoon, the initial hum drum and excitement of school pick up and "what happened at school today" is finished. The house quietens a little as Josh sits down at the kitchen table to do his homework. Sharny needs to call Emma, but wants to ring Jodie too. As she's tiptoeing down the hallway, Josh notices her leaving and says:

"I want $5 for school tomorrow"

By the time she's finished talking to him, she only has time for one phone call. Who does she call?

Is it different?

She changed from Jodie to Emma, didn't she?

How about the conversation she had with Josh? Has it changed from story one to story two?

In our family, the conversation changed from asking why he needed the money, to a lecture on rudeness.

In the first story, Josh tells Sharny that he *needs* $5, in the second story he tells her that he *wants* $5.

But no kid would ever tell their parents that they *want* something. They're way smarter than that, in fact kids are great negotiators, amazing sales people. If a kid really *wants* something, he's not going to tell you that he *wants* it, he's going to change his words. He's going to be much more convincing. He's going to tell you that he *needs* it.

Language is so powerful, if a kid asks you for something they *want*, it's easy to come up with an excuse. But if they ask you for something that they *need*, it's hard not to help them out, they *need* it, right?

When we first realised the power of these words, and the genius of a young child at their use, we were enthralled. Every time Josh would say "I want $5" we would reply with a smart arse comment like "I want a million dollars."

But when he would say "I *need* $5" we would be emotionally bound to ask "what for."

Josh worked this out young, by asking for a *need*, he found an opening. Before long, he just stopped using *want*. And we kept shelling out cash.

Who says adults are smarter than kids?

Back to Emma and Jodie... Why did you change your mind?

Same deal. We just switched the position of *want* and *need*. Go back and read it again. In story one, she *wanted* to call Emma, but *needed* to call Jodie. In story two, she *needed* to call Emma, but only *wanted* to call Jodie.

Pretty powerful stuff, right?

Here's where it gets really interesting...

When we worked this out, we changed our answers. Every time Josh would use *need* on us, we'd ask him "Do you *need* it, or just *want* it?"

If you're a parent, this book just paid for itself, didn't it?

Here it is again, underlined and in bold, so you can find it easily:

Do you *need* it, or just *want* it?

Pretty damn chuffed with ourselves were we, when we worked this out. From then on, we managed to keep a lot more money in the pocket, and had far less arguments steeped in parental guilt, because Josh could work it out for himself.

But wait. Before you go patting us on the back, remember that kids are much smarter than us.

Every time we'd say something like "I can't take you to the skate park, I need to watch the game" we'd get asked; "do you need to watch the game, or just want to?"

That's not all, we found some real beauties. Here are a few, try them on yourself.

"I need a holiday"

"I need a new car"

What about:

"I need sugar in my coffee"

or

"I need milk in my coffee"

or even

"I need coffee"

hmmm... here's a great one:

"I need a drink"

but our all time favourite is this one:

"I need to eat"

Do you *need* to eat, or just *want* to eat? In the 80s, when people with love handles were classed as 'fat', the standard survival guide was that a normal human (without love handles) could go 21 days without food before they would die.

Now, normal (the average) looks more like a rhino than an 80's human, but they swear, 15 minutes after eating half a cow, glued between two loaves of bread and washed down with a litre of cola that they are starving, and they *need* food or they will die!

People need to be honest with themselves, distinguish *want* from *need*. Children *need* everything. Adults grow out of it. If you find yourself saying you *need* something, find out if it is a *need* or just a *want*. Children use *need* on their parents. Don't be so stupid as to use it on yourself.

Mobility, Not Flexibility

immobile - inflexible - mobile - flexible

Do you stretch? If you do, is it best to stretch before or after exercise? Why do you stretch?

If you could sum up an age with one word, you could say 2 would be "no", because "no" is the word most used by the little one who has discovered a sense of self. Early teens would be "awkward," late teens would be "sex" and "alcohol" would be early 20's. Back at age 3, where we both seem to be fairly well stuck, the word would be "why?"

Can you remember when you were a kid how much delicious fun it was asking "why?" to everything? A lot of times we would ask "why?" out of the inbuilt human need for learning, but other times we'd ask "why?" because it was cool to see someone sweat over giving an answer they couldn't, leaving them with one failsafe option: "Because I said so."

We're not much mentally older than 3, and this is probably why we're not welcome at many fitness conventions or seminars. We love to ask "why?" and unwittingly, the answer we get the most is "just because" - it's the fitness industry's equivalent to "because I said so."

One question that can never draw any single, logical stream of thinking is stretching. Athletes have been stretching for years. Drive around early in the morning and you are bound to see a jogger with one foot on a step, leaning over to stretch their hamstrings.

One person will tell you to stretch before you exercise to avoid injury, another will tell you that stretching before exercise will cause injury. One person will tell you that you can't bounce your stretches, and another will tell you that 'dynamic stretching' is the way to go.

So, put your dummy in your mouth, and your bib over your head, think about where you stand in the stretching debate and let's ask "why?"

Why do you stretch?

To avoid injury.

Why?

Because injury is debilitating.

Why?

Because if you injure a muscle, you won't be able to move it.

Why?

blank.

Here's the interesting part. If you injure a muscle, you won't be able to move it. Not necessarily the problem, since it is not the muscle that moves, it is the limb that moves. Engineers will tell you that the muscle moves the limb, but movement happens at the joint.

So, any restricted movement in any joint, is technically an injury. this is important... The joint becomes debilitated. For example, a torn hamstring restricts movement through the knee joint.

A torn hamstring is the reason for the restricted movement, but what is the cause of the torn hamstring. Is it because the hamstring is too tight. What would make it too tight?

Let's get this straight first. Logic dictates that any loss of mobility from normal would be classed as injury. The only thing that matters in an injury then is the degree of debilitation. Is it immobile (cannot move at all), or is it at some varying restricted degree of mobility?

So, why do you stretch?

To avoid injury, to avoid immobility of the joint, or *increase* functional range of motion in the joint to a standard that will mitigate injury.

Why?

Two boxers of exactly the same weight, fitness and ability. Who's going to win the fight? Nine out of ten times, its the guy with the longer reach who's going to win fights.

A greyhound and a dachshund. Who's going to run faster? The

greyhound, because it can go further with each stride.

As humans, we can't compete across species. We've restricted our sport to intra species competition. If we pretest two olympic weight lifters of exactly the same height, weight and reach for primary muscle strength (glutes, hammys, and quads) and they score the exact same strength, is there something else at play when one lifts nearly twice the weight of the other? Of course. I'll tell you what it is in a minute, but first, an experiment.

Go and find yourself a mop, the old fashioned type with long strands of rope. soak it in water until the head is heavy. Now stand it up vertically with the head to the ceiling. Hold the other end with only one hand right at the bottom few inches of the handle.

Now slowly rotate your wrist until the mop is horizontal and feel how hard you have to grip. The further away you get from the vertical plane, the harder it is to grip. Most of the time, anything more than 10 degrees and your wrist strength will fail and the mop will drop.

Now impose this image onto the weightlifters body in full crouch. The head of the mop is representative of the weight above the lifters head. The handle of the mop represents their spine. Your wrist represents your lower back muscles.

The guy who can hold a more upright back will win every time. To the point where an insignificant 5 degree shift in weight can go from easy to impossible. These guys have the exact same anatomy, so why can one keep their back more upright than the other, through the squat movement?

It's not in their lower backs. Slow motion of weight lifters shows that there is little to no movement in the back at all. It's actually in their hip joints. The winning weight lifter is able to open his legs wider, thus changing the mechanics of the lift and reducing the leverage on his lower back. He can do this because he has more mobility through the hip joint.

Why?

The anatomy of the ball and socket hip joint is essentially the same for all humans, it's just that Mr Champion Weight Lifter can move his hip joint like a shoulder joint. Which is how we are meant to move it. If he can do it, so can we.

Why can some people do the splits and others can't? It's got nothing to do with bone restricting bone. It is because of the connective tissue keeping the hip joint in place, one or two of yours and mine are tighter than the weight lifter, or the gymnast, restricting movement in the joint.

Is it even important to be able to do the splits?

This is where it is up to you, and self assessment is the key here. Take a moment to first observe movement in your joints. Do you have full range of motion or are they restricted in some way.

If you find you have restricted functional movement in a joint, you are therefore technically injured, not an acute injury, but very exciting because you have untapped potential.

You don't need to get stronger, you just need to free up the joint so that you have more reach, or less leverage. Work on gaining mobility in that joint, and you can become like the dachshund who finds out he has greyhound legs.

Mobility is the second tier in our athletic pyramid after nutrition. When we see an athlete with a problem that is not nutritionally based, the next logical step for us, before strength, power, fitness or endurance, is mobility.

We're constantly surprised at the difference in performance when an athlete stretches to increase his or her mobility, rather than 'just because'.

It's Just A Game

Like the Colosseum on a public holiday, Suncorp Stadium is deserted. Not a soul in sight. The normal hubbub of the city blocked by thick walls of concrete, the battle ground sits silent. Dormant. High in the stands, barely visible to the resident doves sits a man so still he is forgotten.

The quiet cooing of the doves echoes the sadness of the place. The sadness of the man. Slowly raising his head, hand prints can be seen around his temple. Eyes blinking away the darkness, he looks blankly over the field.

Chest emptying a deep breath he drops his head back into his hands. The sound of his cap falling echoes quietly across the stands. The family of pigeons, tired of one another, take flight into the grey sky, leaving behind one lonely feather, drifting ever so slowly down to earth.

The deep steel eyes of the man focus mindlessly on the feather. He's sitting up now, watching the feather finish it's final flight. As it drifts peacefully down to the field, he thinks about his life, he thinks about the decisions that have led him here.

As the feather makes its last desperate lunge toward heaven, he contemplates the enormity of it all. Slowly, slowly, the feather gives up, and tumbles gently down to it's final resting place.

Staring through the feather, eyes tired, head pounding, he lets his mind wander. He thinks about Robbie Deans, arguably the most consistent rugby coach in history. The master tactician would be at home right now, preparing for the World Cup next year. He's a good man, old Robbie, taking on the job of coaching Australia against his home country of New Zealand. A Brave man.

"I wonder if any of my players will make his team." thinks Ewen. He knows that it's very unlikely. The only player who might had already transferred to another franchise, leaving him with a slew of young school boys and a few tired old war horses to work with.

"I don't blame Berrick," thinks Ewen, "he's at the prime of his career, next year will be his last chance to play at a World Cup. It's hard to stand out when your team has finished bottom three for the past 6 years."

"Reds," he thinks to himself. "What does it mean to those poor players each year. They're the laughing stock of the state. In an era of dominance for Queensland Rugby League, this Union team can't win a game."

"It's not fun anymore. The crowds have thinned, many have turned to league. Home games felt like away games last year. More supporters turned out for the opposition than for my boys."

"Boys" he thinks. "They're just boys." The corners of his mouth start to lift as the players begin filtering onto the field. Dancing, joking, mucking around, they're not yet tamed by the expectations and pressures of professional athletes.

He thinks back to yesterday when he slammed them with hours of torturous fitness and skills practice. He had unleashed a tidal wave of frustration on them, he wanted to break them, to make them his. If they were going to lose again, he didn't want it on their conscience. Like a humble father, he had prepared himself to take the blame. "they're only boys" he thinks again.

Too tired to get up, he watches, unnoticed in the stands.

5 minutes go by. Like a pot put on the stove, he can feel himself start to tremble. On the field the boys have split themselves into teams and are playing touch. "They're so happy," he thinks, deciding to wait a little longer before he has to bring down the hammer of discipline.

Like the pot, he begins to tremble, first in his toes, then his foot, then his legs. On the field, he's watching something take shape, he can feel it forming in his mind.

His feet rattling on the concrete, Ewen's idea becomes clearer. As one of his boys crosses the line for a try, surrounded by whoops and cheers from his mates, on both sides of the field, he loses control.

A triumphant roar of laughter explodes out of his mouth, freezing everyone on the field instantly. He laughs even harder as the comedy of it sets in. When he was a boy, he used to laugh so hard he'd get the giggles. "It's been a long time since I've giggled," he thinks, the puzzled looks on the faces pushing him closer to the edge.

His infectious laughter spreads. By the time he reaches the field, some of the players are on their backs. "My God, it feels good to laugh like this" he thinks. Clearly, some of the players feel the same way, like a wraith, the weight of defeat from the older players drifts into the now bright Queensland sky.

"Boys... Men..." he booms, face flushed with pride.

"Take away the money, take away the competition, take away the crowds and you're left with just rugby. Rugby is a game. Just a game..."

The boys have crowded him now, they can sense something great is happening, their faces light up with expectation as their new coach continues.

"A game is meant to be fun," he continues.

"This season, we're going to bring that back. Winning may be the number one priority for every other team, but for us, we're going to have fun."

Mumbles of excitement building up in his team, he quickly carries on.

"Life is too short to not have fun, if you think you cannot enjoy yourself playing rugby for the Queensland Reds, then you owe it to yourself to find something else, something that you can love, something you do enjoy, something that brings you fun."

"It is our duty to ourselves, to each other, to our State and to the world, we must bring fun back into sport. Fun at our level of the game will give permission to younger kids to have fun."

"Watching you play touch before reminded me why I love the game. Watching you play touch is far more entertaining than watching any game of professional rugby for the past 10 years. While everybody else is getting stricter and stricter, cogs in a big machine; we will become unpredictable, we will play like kids in the back yard. We will have fun. Win, lose or draw, we *will* have fun!"

And have fun they did. From a 6 year losing streak, with a team of unknowns, Ewen McKenzie and the Queensland Reds played a remarkable, unpredictable game of rugby. Every single week they entertained the growing crowds. Previously embarrassed supporters came out in hoards. Home games became a sell out.

Rugby, arguably a dying, over complicated sport with stifling rules became exciting again. the old institutions scoffed, "you can't play like that," while their own children put down their game station remotes, preferring the back yards, yelling names like Digby, Radike, Quade or Genia.

One by one the mightiest teams fell to the unpredictable, exciting, entertaining brand of rugby McKenzie's boys brought onto the park.

Just over 12 months after the speech, James Horwill, captain of the youngest team to ever play Super rugby held the cup above his head, surrounded by a deafening roar of the sell out home crowd.

Sport, just like life is just a game. And games are meant to be fun. If you can't find joy and pleasure in your job, your marriage, your sport, your life.... change it. You deserve to have fun - because if you focus on fun, you can never lose.

Climb

In the closing days of the 2012 London Olympics, the first lap of the women's 800 metre final is being run. The competitors are all bunched together, jogging. Nobody is racing, nobody wants to take the lead. 800 metres is only 2 laps of the track, normally run at a near sprint. Astoundingly, these women are barely breaking stride.

The commentators are shocked, the crowd doesn't like it. As the bell goes for the second and final lap, they try to will them on, giving them energy, shouting at them, pleading them to just *compete*.

But they don't.

Finally, with only 200m to go, the competitors seem to break out of their haze and sprint. It is a pitiful end, the women have left it too late, the world and olympic records have long passed, and every one of them crosses the line to their slowest official times ever.

The commentators struggle to hide their disgust, but the stadium crowd doesn't care. People can be seen getting up from their seats, angry that they had to witness this embarrassment to sport.

Humans love watching people perform at their best, it crosses political boundaries and language barriers. People all over the world get a lump in their throats when they watch the likes of Mo Farah, willing himself to the line with a battered, exhausted body, or watching Usain Bolt, thundering down the track for what we all hope will be another world record.

Athletes inspire us to try a little harder in our own lives.

So when they put in a lacklustre performance, like the women in the 800m finals, we get offended. It's not *right*, it's not *just*. It's *cheating*, people say. And it is. The competitors have been cheated out of a real race, the winner has been cheated out of being crowned a real champion and the audience has been cheated out of a chance to be inspired.

Is *your* performance any different?

Is it OK for you to hold back from performing at *your* best? Is it OK for you to be *uninspiring*.

People think that competition is cruel, but it's not. Non-competition is cruel. When you underperform to protect the feelings of the people around you, it's patronising and offensive.

Nobody benefits if you perform at anything less than your best. Underperformance doesn't help you, and it doesn't help them.

This goes for more than just exercise. Work, sport, family, career, love, dieting. Everything you do should be done to the best of your abilities. Because even if you're not at the front of the pack, you're in front of somebody. And if you're in front of someone, they are watching you, and you are therefore *leading* them.

Never hold back, always give your best performance. Demand that the people ahead of you do the same.

We've all tried helping the people in the cave, but it hasn't worked, they keep trying to make us one of them.

It's time to turn your back, face the sun and climb. One day soon, when your joyous, unconfined spirit lights up the dark, they will follow.

FITlosophy 2

Embracing Excellence in a World of Mediocrity

What is the potential for human performance, when we are not held back by feelings of unease, guilt?

What will the world be like, when fit, which is the direct opposite of unhealthy, takes a stand. When the leaders turn their backs and the gap is opened. When excellence is the norm, and athletes realise they are born for inspiration, not excuses.

Is it even possible, or are we living a pipe dream, a fantasy? Is excellence pointless, is it a scam?

Fitlosophy 2 goes there. More hard hitting, more intriguing and more thought provoking. If you liked this book, then you'll love the sequel. Be sure not to miss it.

To be notified when Fitlosophy 2 becomes available, register your interest right now at:

sharnyandjulius.com/fitlosophy2

Never Diet Again

Escape the Diet Trap Forever

Everyone who has been to university will agree that hands on work experience has taught them way more than the books and lecturers ever did, or ever could. Old style teaching simply doesn't work. What *does* work is self education; experience based learning.

People need to learn things for themselves.

Our first book, *Never Diet Again*, is exactly that! A treasure trove of experiments and strategies for you to try. A cleverly laid out pathway that guides you to a healthier lifestyle... Not by rote learning, but by experience.

If, after reading *FITlosophy*, you feel ready to start climbing, but don't know where to start, then *Never Diet Again* is your roadmap. If you have been robbed and confused by too many conflicting messages; from marketing companies, junk food companies or diet companies, then *Never Diet Again* will clear the path and light the way.

It will start you on the journey you've been looking for. A journey that will change the way you see your body forever!

You can find out more by going to

www.sharnyandjulius.com/neverdietagain

About the Authors

Sharny and Julius

Renegade fitness experts Sharny and Julius shot to stardom very quickly when their first book, *Never Diet Again* was released to the public in June 2011. The book was an adaptation of their step by step *escape the diet trap* program they created for their private clients. So successful was the program in changing people's lives that the clients literally begged Sharny and Julius to make it into a book, which would be more accessible to friends and relatives overseas.

After the release of *Never Diet Again*, the couple realised that while very successful, it was just another weight loss solution in a sea of thousands, if not millions of solutions. But people as a whole were still getting "fatter and sicker".

After much soul searching and deliberation, they decided that losing weight wasn't the problem. The motivation for losing weight was the problem. Fat and unhealthy was the norm; healthy, athletic people were the minority. The word 'fat' had become offensive. Exercise was too much of a chore.

That's when they decided to write the book *FITlosophy*. In their words, it is "a collection of parables for athletes". But after consuming it, readers agree that it is far more than that. It is a profound set of philosophical viewpoints that cut right to the heart of the human condition. Brutally honest, courageous, confronting, and often humorous, the stories told in this book reveal a part of the human psyche readers didn't even know was there. *FITlosophy* will sit with the reader for a long time after the words have actually been read.

In January 2012, they collaborated with renowned artist Ayesha Henderson to create a children's book that had "beautiful bright pictures and an easy to read, but important message that they could share with their kids". *Where Have All The Pixies Gone?* was released in October 2012.

At the time of publication, Sharny and Julius are writing the sequel to *FITlosophy*, which promises to be their magnum opus, their "greatest gift to humanity". They are regulars on daytime TV, radio and newspapers in their home country of Australia.

The couple are expecting their fourth child in January 2013 and plan on having one more. Sharny is the high energy super mum personality in the couple. Julius' often deep, philosophical nature is contrasted by his wicked sense of humour.

For more information or to contact Sharny and Julius, head to their private website\blog.

www.sharnyandjulius.com